FIGHT x FOOD
DIET AND NUTRITION TO WIN AT LIFE

Fight Food: Diet and Nutrition to Win at Life is published under Erudition, a sectionalized division under Di Angelo Publications, Inc.

Erudition is an imprint of Di Angelo Publications.
Copyright 2024.
All rights reserved.
Printed in the United States of America.

Di Angelo Publications
Los Angeles, California

Library of Congress
Fight Food: Diet and Nutrition to Win at Life
First Edition
ISBN: 978-1-955690-58-4
Paperback

Words: Eric Triliegi
Photography: Viktoria Sirakova
Cover Design: Savina Deianova
Interior Design: Kimberly James
Editor: Willy Rowberry

Downloadable via www.dapbooks.shop and other e-book retailers.

No part of this publication may be reproduced, distributed, or transmitted in any form or by any means without the prior written permission of the publisher, except in the case of brief quotations embodied in critical reviews and certain other noncommercial uses permitted by copyright law. For permission requests, contact info@diangelopublications.com.

For educational, business, and bulk orders, contact distribution@diangelopublications.com.

FIGHT x FOOD

DIET AND NUTRITION TO WIN AT LIFE

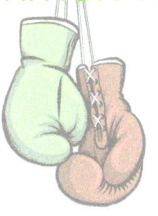

ERIC_TRILIEGI

CELEBRITY NUTRITIONIST & CHEF TO

@thenotoriousmma
@loganpaul
@ksi
@adinross
@kingryan
@calebplant
@taylerholder

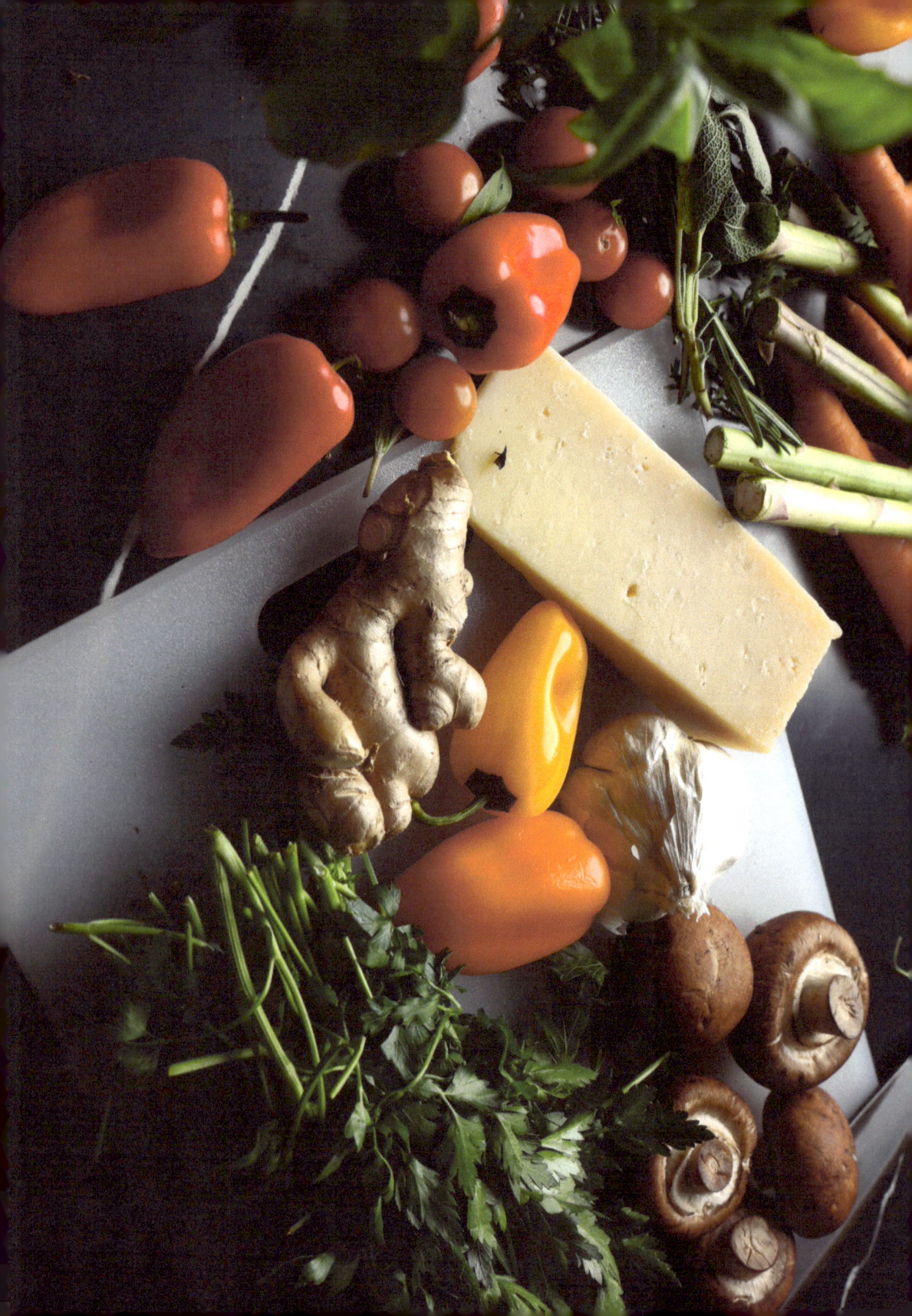

CONTENTS

Foreword ... 11

THE FIGHT

Introduction: Exploring A World Of Flavors ... 15
Humble Beginnings — From Slopes To Stovetops ... 19
Finding My Footing ... 21
The Ultimate Fighter ... 25
Expanding My Passions ... 28
Nurturing Champions, Building Dreams ... 31
Embracing New Horizons In La ... 34
Healing Through Food With Demi Lovato ... 37
The World Of Champions — Mcgregor Vs. Khabib ... 43
A Culinary Knockout — Ksi And The Black Cod Revelation ... 47
Working With Logan Paul ... 52
From Injury To Recovery With Conor Mcgregor ... 55
Embracing New Challenges — Working With Influencer Boxers ... 59

THE FOOD

BREAKFAST

Egg, Mushroom, And Avocado Scramble With Chicken Sausage ... 68
Potato, Onion, And Zucchini Frittata ... 70
Everything Bagel Crusted Salmon Over Arugula Salad ... 72
Simple Egg Scramble With Baby Potatoes, Bell Pepper, And Onion ... 74

Egg And Goat Cheese Scramble With Veggies 75
Avocado Toast With Eggs, Cherry Tomatoes, And Spinach 77
Crêpes With Fresh Fruit Compote And Over Easy Eggs 78
Fried Egg Sandwich With Avocado, Sriracha, Mayo, And Micro Greens 80
Breakfast Banana Pancakes, Eggs And Chives 81

MAIN COURSES

Shrimp And Garlic Pasta 86
Avocado Chicken Salad 87
Chicken Pasta Salad 88
Salmon Poke 90
Pan Seared Oven Finished Salmon With Roasted Veggies 92
Broccoli With Beef 94
Orange Chicken Over Quinoa 96
Healthy Turkey Chili 98
Salmon Cakes 99
Quinoa And Squash Salad With Cranberries, Pecans, And Pears 100
Steak And Eggs With Chili Verde 102
Lasagna 104

SIGNATURE DISHES

Lovato N' Lime 109
Ksi Black Cod Over Jasmine Rice 113
Logan Paul's Butter Noodles With Baked Herb Chicken Breast 117
DK Salmon 119
Conor's Chops 123
Patrick's Curry 127

SNACKS

Overnight Chia Cups	132
Caprese Sliders With Balsamic	133
Paleo Blueberry Muffins	134
Chicken Satay And Peanut Sauce	136
Bagels And Lox (Smoked Salmon Bagel)	138
Blueberry Compote Parfait	139
Cucumber Salad	140
Fruit Smoothie	141
Cauliflower Fried Rice	143
Spicy Roasted Chickpeas	145
Almond Butter Balls	147
Avocado Chocolate Mousse	148

SMOOTHIES

Green Smoothie Bowl	153
Cocoa Almond Protein Smoothie	155
Oatmeal Breakfast Smoothie	156
Rehydration Smoothie	157
Caramel Protein Shake	158
Chocolate Covered Strawberry Smoothie	158

CUT WEIGHT QUICK LIKE A PRO

MACROS

THANK YOU

PUBLISHER'S NOTE

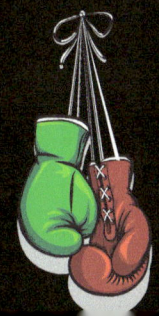

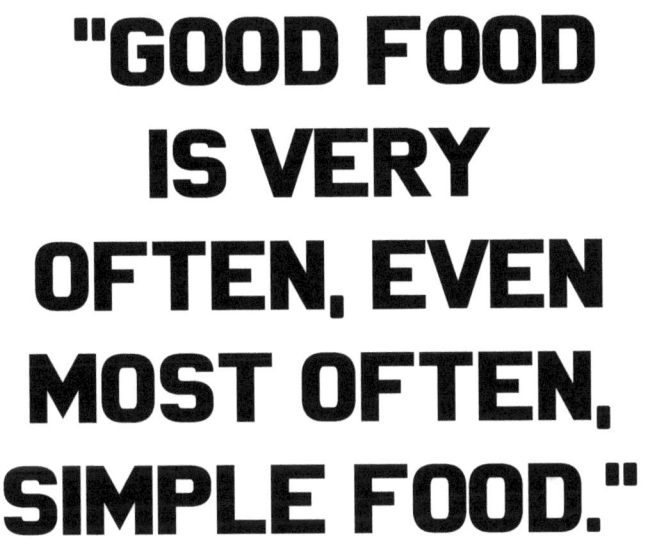

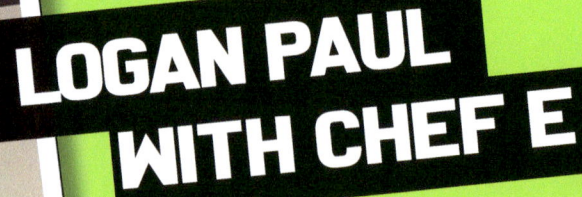

LOGAN PAUL WITH CHEF E

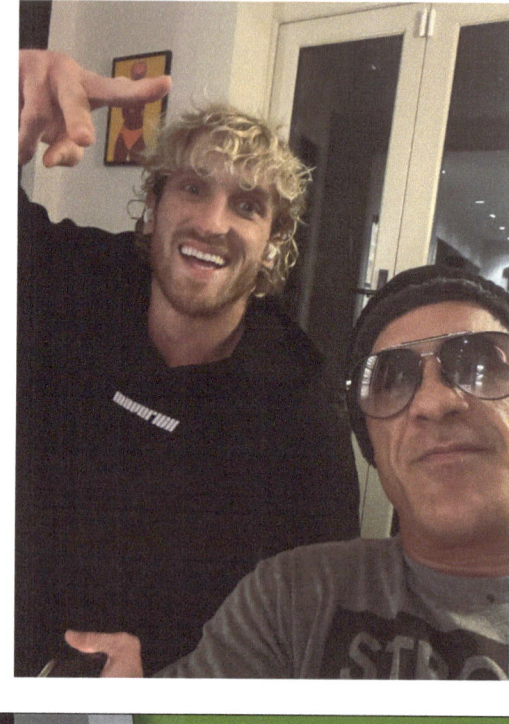

I needed a fight, chef. Not just a regular chef, but someone who knew nutrition as well as cooking delicious food.

FOREWORD

by Logan Paul, professional wrestler

I first heard about Chef E when we he was working with my rival at the time: KSI. I heard he made pretty good food, and at the time, I knew I needed a fight chef. Not just a regular chef, but someone who knew nutrition as well as being able to cook delicious food. I knew Chef E was the guy.

If you haven't heard about him, Chef E has cooked for a lot of the biggest fighters in the world. I was happy to get him on my team—or should I say, I was lucky enough to get him on my team.

Working with Chef E means that no camp has been a struggle for me. Even when I'm cutting weight, I never feel like I'm suffering. It's everything that you need to succeed. I come out of the camp feeling great, strong, and ready. A large part of that is because of what I'm putting in my body.

I've tried a lot of chefs, and out of all the chefs I've had, Chef E is hands down the best. The ingredients are simple but effective. He doesn't overcook. The food is clean, delicious, and gets the job done.

At this point, we have now done three fight camps together, and we have worked together outside of camp as well. His food is exactly what you need as a fighter, and I greatly appreciate that.

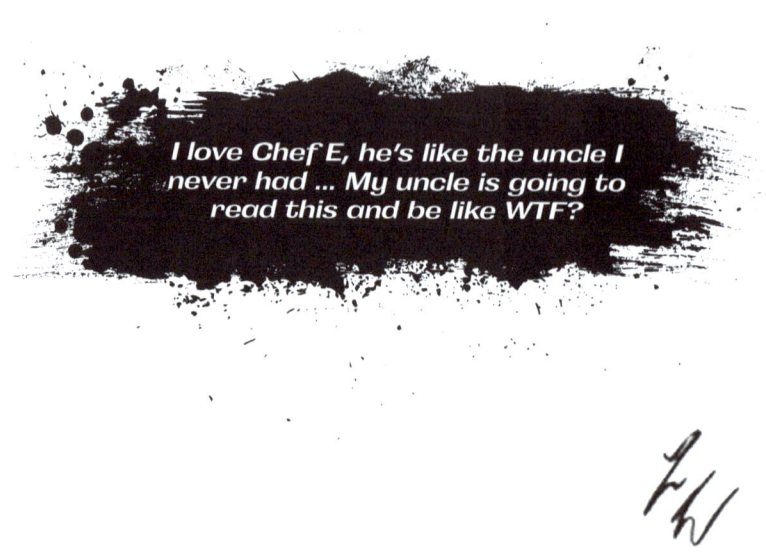

I love Chef E, he's like the uncle I never had ... My uncle is going to read this and be like WTF?

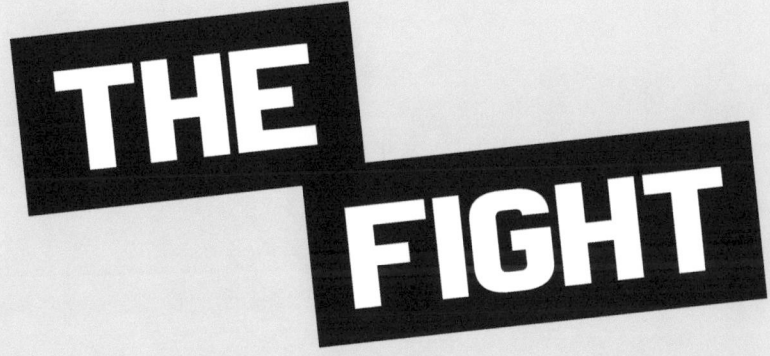

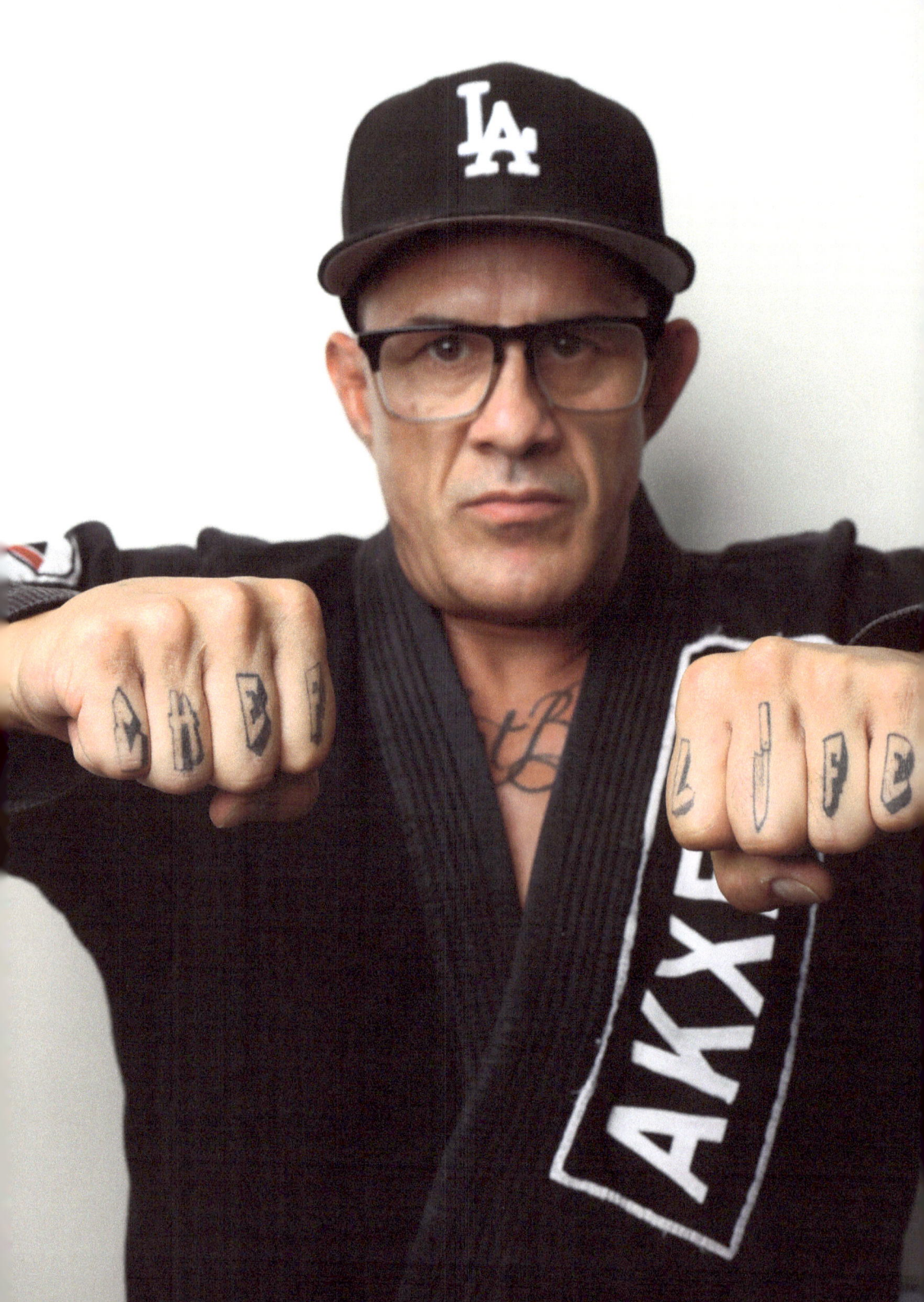

INTRODUCTION
Exploring a World of Flavors

In the culinary world, I've become known as a nutritional chef, blending my love for food and nutrition. This has always been my passion, and I have put in consistent and steadfast effort into getting to this point in my career. When I was younger, there were also a surprising number of encounters and opportunities presented to me that have all led me to the path that I'm on now.

My mother raised me in Lake Tahoe, and the two of us had to navigate the challenges in our lives together. We weren't the most well off, and had very limited resources, but I had a natural curiosity towards food. Even as a child, I would do what I could to liven up our meals. I'd experiment with Top Ramen, adding different ingredients and flavors to make it more interesting.

I remember my first eye-opening encounter with the world of gastronomy, and it happened when I was still a kid. My friend Andrea Villaret introduced me to his dad's French restaurant, Chez Villaret. We had gone into the kitchen to watch the chefs prepare the food, and I witnessed firsthand what went into creating all different types of cuisine. This experience sparked a fascination with food that has stayed with me until now.

Later, around the age of eleven or twelve, my birthday wish was to try something new — sushi. This was the late '80s, and sushi was still relatively unfamiliar to many.

The Japanese restaurant's ambiance with bamboo and koi fish curtains made it seem like a magical place. The kind Japanese lady who owned the place introduced me to the world of sushi, allowing me to sample various fish types and the fresh wasabi, which left a lasting impression on my young palate. An enduring friendship with the restaurant owner, Seiko, grew over the years. She became my mentor, teaching me about Japanese cuisine, sushi preparation, and the importance of selecting quality ingredients.

Throughout my teenage years, I continued exploring food from different regions and trying new flavors. I began cooking my own dishes and even started experimenting with preparing Japanese cuisine.

As I entered my twenties, my passion for food continued to evolve. I honed my culinary skills, seeking out unique and diverse experiences. I dove into nose-to-tail cooking, experimenting with various cuts of meat, and played around with flavor combinations, pushing away from what was more common.

The desire to understand nutrition's impact on athletic performance led me to expand my knowledge of nutrition and incorporate that into my cooking. This unique blend of skills set me apart in the industry, allowing me to cater to fighters during their fight camps and weight cuts.

When working with my clients, I take pride in educating them about the foods they consume. To start, I tell them that their meal is very clean — which is something I ensure in every meal I make for my fighters — and then go into more detail. From explaining the nutritional components of each dish to where the ingredients are sourced, I aim to make their experience insightful and enjoyable.

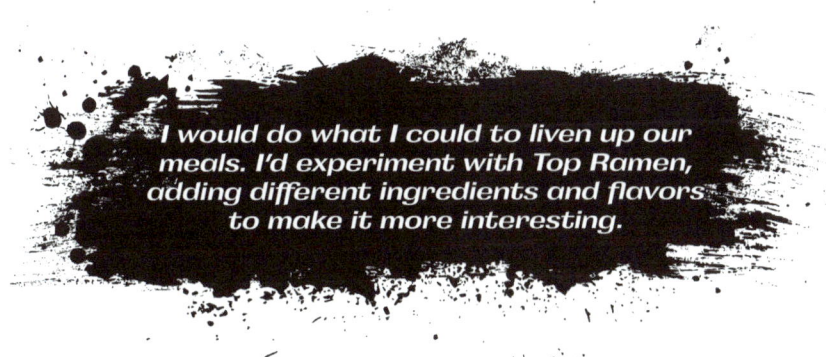

I would do what I could to liven up our meals. I'd experiment with Top Ramen, adding different ingredients and flavors to make it more interesting.

My life's journey as a chef and nutritionist has been shaped by my past — with my humble beginnings and the relationships I was able to build throughout it. Being able to pursue my passion starting from such a young age has enabled me to hone my skills throughout the years and focus on a specific set of needs. A large part of my career is dedicated to providing flavorful and nourishing meals to support the athletic journeys of my clients, and through this, I get the daily thrill of creating delectable and healthy dishes.

I invite you to join me as I reflect on my formative days. The coming chapters hold stories of triumphs, challenges, and the mentorship that played vital roles in my culinary pursuits. Let's explore together the diverse and delicious tapestry of flavors that have been woven into my life.

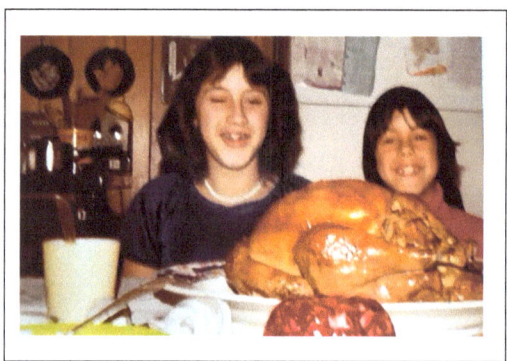

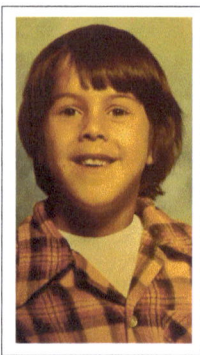

Eric. Eric (right) and sister Tina celebrating Thanksgiving in Lake Tahoe.

CHAPTER 1

Humble Beginnings — From Slopes to Stovetops

My journey into the culinary world started in the beautiful surroundings of Lake Tahoe. My passion was ignited when I was only a child, and my dreams were encouraged mainly by my mentor, Seiko, and other supportive figures in my life. I started on the right path because of them, but unfortunately, I wasn't able to stay on course.

During my teenage years, around the age of sixteen, my focus on food and my other priorities waned. Growing up with a single mom, life wasn't easy. We didn't have a lot of money, and it was hard for my mom to remain present in my life and also provide us with what we needed. She tried her best, but still lacked control over my choices. Consequently, I fell into the grip of a severe drug problem, leading to periods of incarceration.

Around this time, there were other interests that I sought to pursue. My friends and I were determined to ski without breaking the bank. So, we came up with a plan: we'd work at different places to get free ski passes.

During our snow-filled adventures, I stumbled

upon a great opportunity at the Governor's Restaurant, high up in Heavenly Valley. Besides getting to ski for free, they offered me a chance to try my hand at cooking. I may have exaggerated a bit on my job application, claiming I was an experienced line cook, but they hired me for the position anyway.

The first day in the restaurant's kitchen was a mix of nerves and excitement. The place was buzzing with activity, and it was obvious I had limited cooking experience. But my boss, a laid-back type who fit right into Tahoe's bohemian vibe, saw potential in me. Instead of turning me away, he decided to mentor me and help me grow as a chef. He taught me the basics, like grilling steaks and preparing pasta, gradually building my confidence.

As the weeks went by, I perfected the dishes my boss had taught me, and grilling became my specialty. The restaurant, surrounded by Tahoe's artistic and natural charm, became a haven for my exploration, and it reignited the spark I had when I was younger. I was drawn back into the kitchen, becoming immersed in learning everything I could in this restaurant.

This short gig turned out to be a life-changing experience that helped draw me away from my old lifestyle. I distanced myself from old habits and bad influences — both mentally, and physically. After rounding off my job at the Governor's Restaurant, I relocated to Santa Rosa.

CHAPTER 2
Finding My Footing

After relocating, I took some time to discover what it is I really wanted to do with my life. My passion for cooking had been pivotal before, but there had been no direction in it. As I took some time to move forward with any solid career plans, I took on several odd jobs in the meantime.

From my time cooking, both as a job previously and as an ongoing hobby, I had taken an interest in the relationship between my health and the food that I consumed. More specifically, I paid specific attention to the ingredients that went into my meals, and their nutritional value. I decided to learn more about the direct impact nutrition played in people's bodies and health.

My newfound interest in nutrition and its impact on the body naturally progressed into learning more by taking various courses, including functional movement, exercise, and Olympic powerlifting. When I became a personal trainer, I integrated nutrition into my training programs.

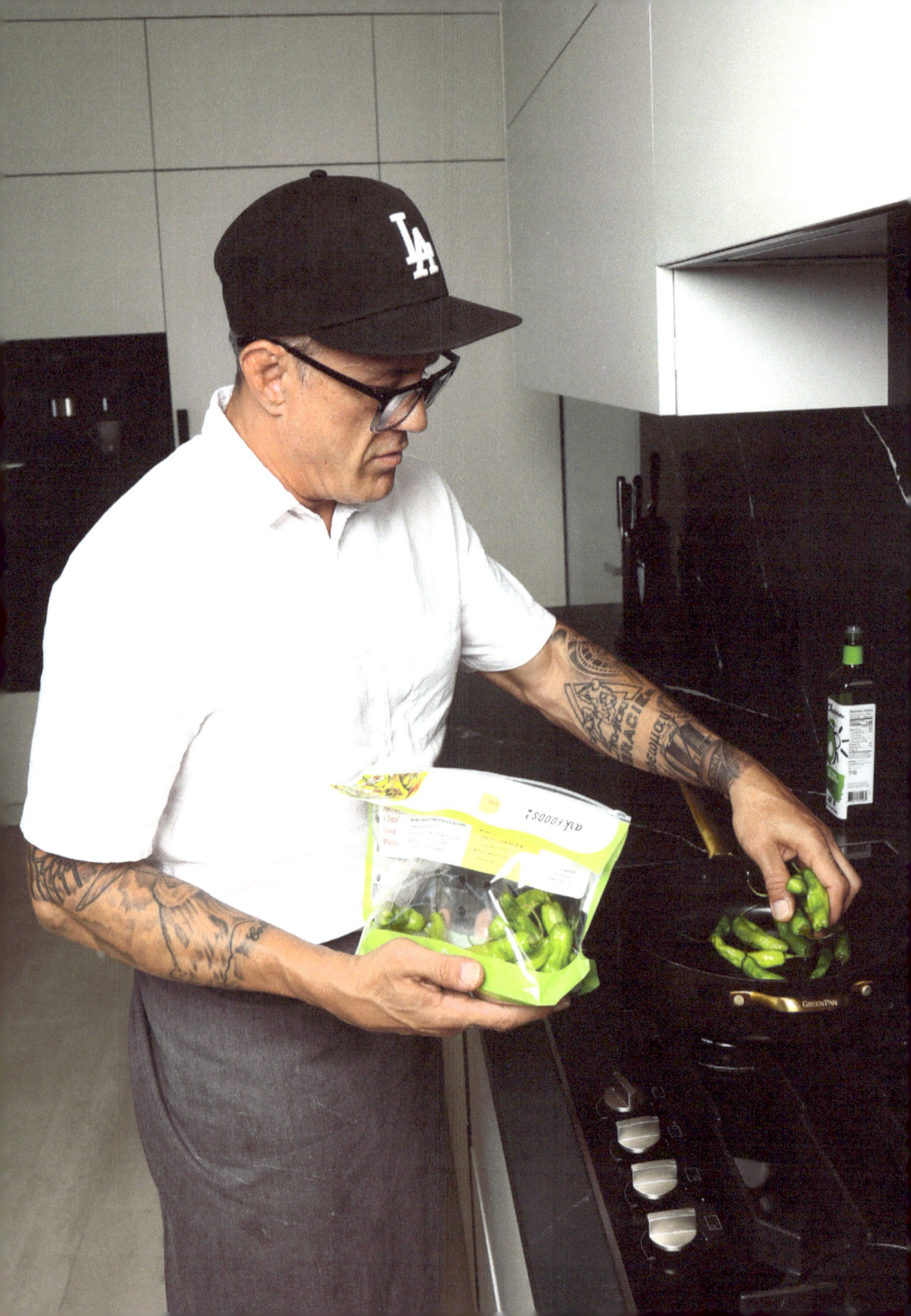

Starting as a personal trainer gave me a natural segue into the world of athletes. Though I had never been part of a team sport, I had a natural inclination towards solo activities like snowboarding, skiing, and skateboarding, so this realm wasn't completely foreign to me. I knew of the physical demand that sports had, and I curated meal plans to best suit my clients, regardless of the sport they participated in.

As I delved deeper into the world of sports nutrition, an opportunity to work with NBA clients from the Sacramento Kings presented itself. Hungry for success, I was willing to do whatever it took to secure a prominent client, even if it meant sleeping in my car just to be close to their homes. Determined to be available at a moment's notice, I went to Sacramento and stayed there, living out of run-down motels and making sacrifices that only a passionate dream-chaser would understand.

With persistence and resilience, I began making strides, and my clientele started growing. Among the first prominent athletes I worked with was Miesha Tate, a formidable fighter known in the Strikeforce world. Her trust in me allowed me to take charge of her strength conditioning and nutrition throughout her camp. When she secured the Strikeforce world title with a dominant submission victory, I felt an overwhelming sense of accomplishment and knew I was on the right path.

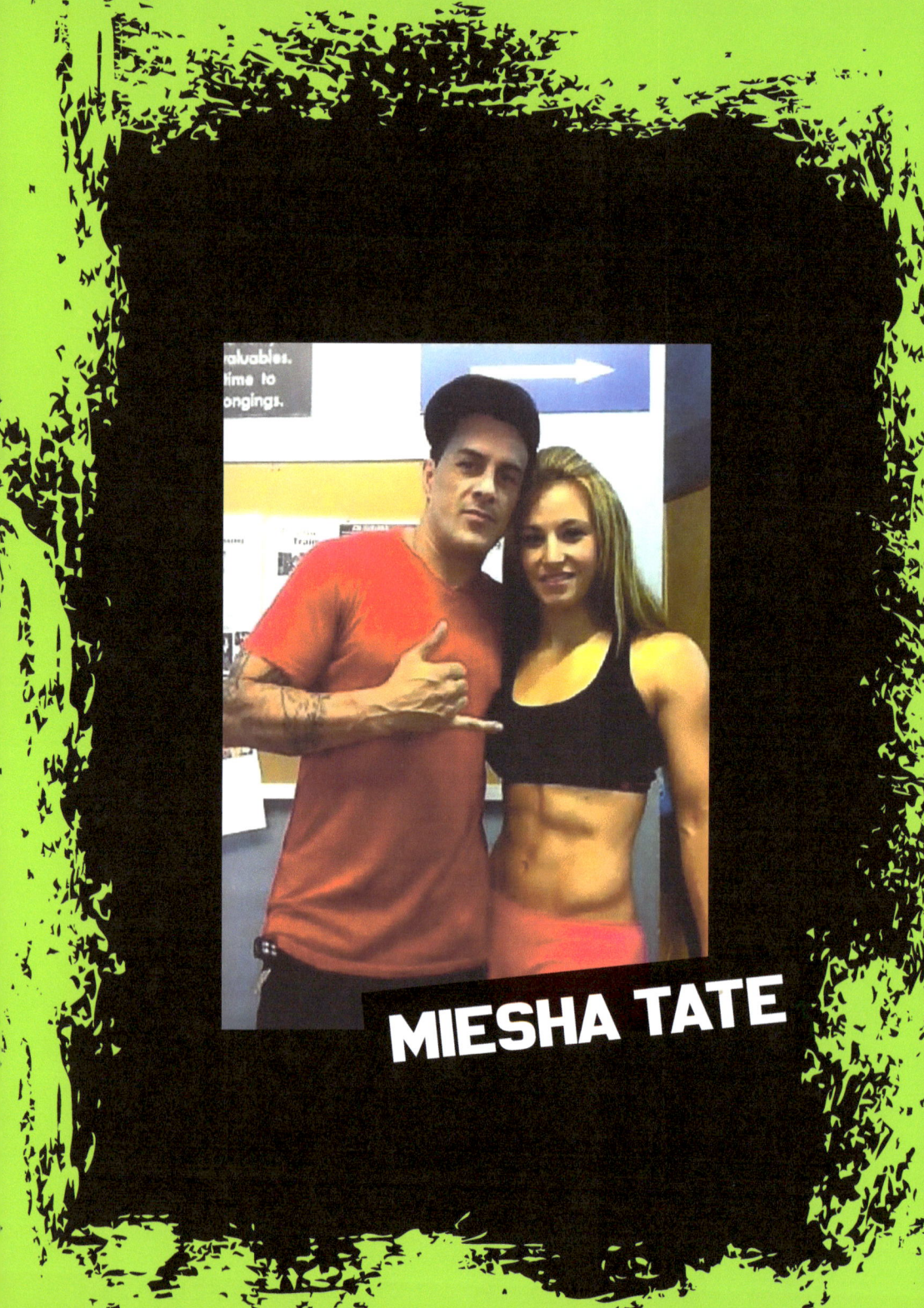

CHAPTER 3
The Ultimate Fighter

As word spread about my expertise, more fighters sought my guidance. Anthony Pettis, a popular UFC fighter, reached out after hearing of Miesha's success. We embarked on a remarkable journey together, as we honed his skills both inside and outside the cage. Anthony's triumphs under my guidance, including winning a UFC world title, further solidified my reputation in the fighting world.

Every big client I took on led me further and further into the world of fighting, and I took strides into becoming a specialized and unique nutritionist. I would provide my fighters with personalized training and nutritional support, but one of the unusual choices I made was allowing fighters, who had come in from different places, to live with me. Dustin from Kansas City and a few fighters from Japan were among the first to join me. However, it was a young kid named Chris Holdsworth who made the most significant impact.

Chris was a force of nature, and his dedication and skill in jiu-jitsu were extraordinary. He quickly became an asset to our team. I offered him a place to live, covering his training, food, and other necessities. As Chris settled in, he tried out for The Ultimate Fighter show, a reality series offering promising fighters the chance to win a contract with the UFC. In a way that felt almost fated, I was also invited to be a coach in the same season.

Chris ended up joining my team on the show, and it was a proud moment for both of us. His grit and hard work paid off as he went on to win the Ultimate Fighter, earning a contract with the UFC.

My experience with the show also proved to be invaluable. The Ultimate Fighter provided an excellent platform to train and guide young fighters. The show's format allowed them to live together, experience victories and defeats, and develop strong teamwork and camaraderie — and I was beside them throughout it all.

To ensure that I could offer the best support for the fighters, I meticulously gathered information from each of them, including their preferences, dislikes, allergies, and dietary restrictions. Understanding their eating habits and favorite cuisines helped me tailor their meals and create an optimal nutrition plan.

To further enhance my understanding of their health, I encouraged them to undergo blood tests to assess vital markers. This valuable insight allowed me to craft personalized nutrition plans that optimized their performance and well-being. These experiences were yet another step in my deepening the understanding of the role nutrition plays in everyone's lives, and I was able to take this knowledge and integrate it into the foundation of my work.

Although I was satisfied with my single season in The Ultimate Fighter, I was met with a delightful surprise when my client, Anthony Pettis, took on the role of coach on the show in a subsequent season. It was an honor to be invited to assist him once again during the exciting Season 20. I found myself reliving the excitement of the show, but this time from a different perspective, as I worked side by side with Anthony in his coaching role.

To add to the thrill, another one of my clients, Carla Esparza, also participated in that season of The Ultimate Fighter. I had been diligently taking care of her nutrition and weight cutting for the show, and witnessing her emerge victorious was a moment of immense pride for me. It was a testament to the hard work we had put in together, and it reinforced my belief in the power of dedication and discipline.

Overall, my time on the show throughout both seasons was something that helped guide me i, and I look back at the time with great pride.

CHAPTER 4
Expanding My Passions

Working with Chris Holdsworth, both as my client as a mentee on The Ultimate Fighter, opened a new area of interest for me in my late twenties, and I found myself drawn to the world of jiu jitsu. Under the guidance of remarkable mentors like David Terrell and Cesar Gracie, I immersed myself in this dynamic martial art. Terrell, my first teacher, was a force to be reckoned with, a true master of American Jiu-Jitsu. His impeccable record and unparalleled skills left an indelible mark on me.

Over the past 25 years, jiu jitsu has been a steadfast companion in my life. Training with remarkable fighters like Terrell, Jake Shields, Gilbert Melendez, Uriah Faber, and Dustin Barry blessed me with invaluable experiences. The vibrant jiu jitsu community opened doors for me, allowing me to work with fighters, both nurturing their bodies with the right nutrition and crafting dishes to fuel their training camps.

As my focus shifted towards jiu jitsu, I delved deeper into understanding performance foods and food science. I became fascinated by the intricate ways food interacts with the body. Questions like how a carrot affects athletic performance or the impact of certain compounds on insulin spikes intrigued me. My quest to comprehend food's role in fueling the human body wasn't confined to the gym; it extended to the kitchen.

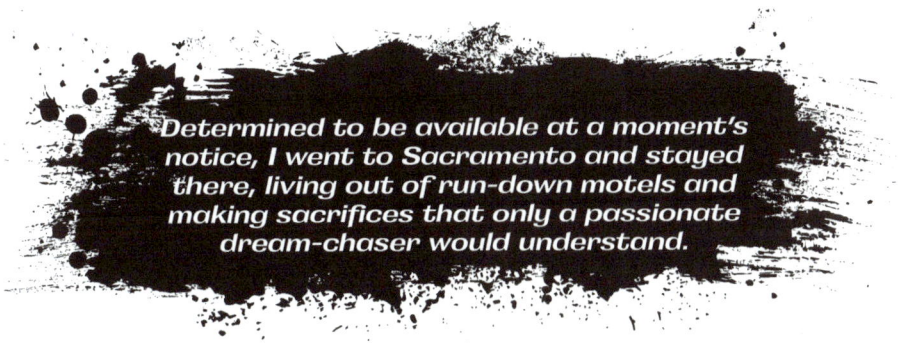

Determined to be available at a moment's notice, I went to Sacramento and stayed there, living out of run-down motels and making sacrifices that only a passionate dream-chaser would understand.

Expanding my learning wasn't limited to formal classrooms. While I did take some classes in my mid-twenties, I realized that traditional schooling wasn't my preferred route. Instead, I became a dedicated self-educator, immersing myself in countless studies, voraciously reading and learning. I stayed updated on the latest fad diets, continually researching the ever-evolving food industry to discern the best choices for my clients. My focus extended to sourcing ethically produced ingredients, supporting organic farms, and understanding the impact of pesticides and hormones on food quality.

The art of cooking, too, became my canvas of exploration. From the age of 25 onwards, I cooked passionately for others, honing my culinary skills.

My extensive travels for work provided me with invaluable opportunities to work with diverse chefs from around the world. The exposure to different cuisines, techniques, and flavors enriched my culinary repertoire. However, my most profound learning moments took place within the walls of my own kitchen, where I engaged in countless trials and errors, discovering the harmonies and contradictions of flavors.

My journey has been marked by self-reliance and an insatiable hunger to succeed. Raised in a single-parent household, I learned to rely on myself from an early age. This independence shaped me into a self-made chef and nurtured a self-starter spirit within me. Throughout my life, I never shied away from challenges, continuously seeking to carve my own path in the culinary world.

As I reflect on my experiences, I embrace the realization that my journey has been a beautiful tapestry of self-discovery. The passion for food, the love for jiu jitsu, and the dedication to understanding nutrition have intertwined to shape the chef I am today. My culinary adventures are a testament to the power of self-motivation, the joy of lifelong learning, and the profound impact of nurturing both the body and the soul through food.

CHAPTER 5
Nurturing Champions, Building Dreams

In the more immediate aftermath of The Ultimate Fighter, I found myself back in Sacramento, eager to see what the future held. I realized that my career had taken on a fascinating duality. On one hand, I was deeply involved in the world of mixed martial arts, working with talented fighters, guiding them on their paths to greatness, and sharing their triumphs and defeats. On the other hand, my love for food and culinary arts was blossoming into something extraordinary.

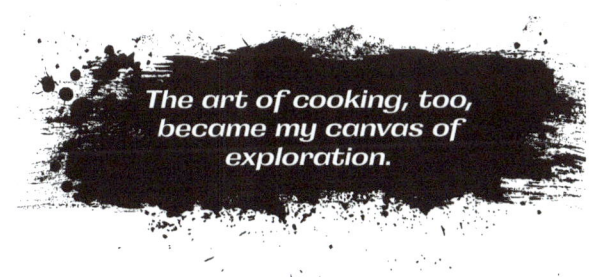

The art of cooking, too, became my canvas of exploration.

During my time back home, I crossed paths with another rising star in the fighting world — Tiffany Van, a fierce and dynamic stand-up fighter with formidable skills in Muay Thai. Impressed by her talent and dedication, I became her manager and took on the responsibility of overseeing her nutrition and dietary needs. It was a perfect blend of my two passions, and I was excited to see where this new collaboration would lead us.

Tiffany and I formed an incredible team, and our journey together took us on thrilling adventures, including a trip to Amsterdam and the Netherlands. There, she competed and secured the prestigious Lion Fight world title, not once but twice! The victories we celebrated together were like sweet rewards for the hard work and commitment we poured into every aspect of her training and nutrition.

But life in the fast-paced world of mixed martial arts never stood still for too long. Just as Tiffany was achieving greatness in the ring, I found myself being called back to Las Vegas. Anthony Pettis was gearing up for a significant UFC world title defense against the formidable Hayfield. The stakes were

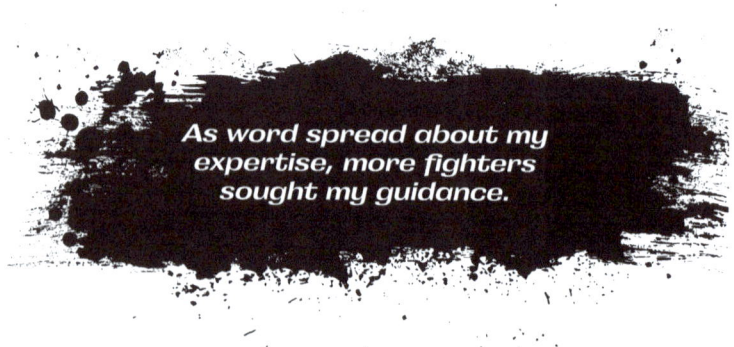

As word spread about my expertise, more fighters sought my guidance.

high, and as his trusted chef and nutritionist, I knew I had to be there to support him in every way possible.

Our fight camp was set up in Milwaukee, where Anthony and his brother called home. It was a familiar place for me too, as my family roots traced back to this city. I took this opportunity to revisit places that held precious memories from my childhood, embracing the nostalgia of those cherished times.

This chapter in my life was a rollercoaster of emotions, with its highs and lows, victories and defeats. Through it all, I learned to appreciate the sweet taste of triumph and to endure the bitter moments of failure. My passion for the culinary arts also continued to grow, as I experimented with flavors and learned through the process of trial and error.

With a heart full of determination and a passion for both fighting and food, I step forward into the unknown, eager to explore the boundless possibilities that await me. Each day brings fresh insights into the art of cooking and the science of nutrition, and I revel in the journey of self-discovery, both in and out of the ring. As the world of mixed martial arts continues to captivate me, I find myself more convinced than ever that my true calling lies in nurturing the bodies and souls of fighters through the power of nourishment.

CHAPTER 6

Embracing New Horizons in LA

As I continued to work and form new connections, I had to make a big decision about what would be best for me moving forward — I decided to move to LA. One of the main reasons for the move was to be closer to my clients. I had cultivated strong relationships with many fighters and athletes in Southern California, and living there allowed me to be more hands-on in their training and nutrition. Being in close proximity meant I could be on top of their progress, ensuring they stayed on track with their weight and fitness goals.

Living in LA opened up a world of opportunities for me. It was a city buzzing with activity and was a hub for the entertainment industry. As my reputation as a skilled chef and nutritionist grew, I found myself branching out into different aspects of Hollywood. I had the chance to work with some actors, and my client list expanded to include some prominent names like Demi Lovato and the Lee Iacocca family.

The move to LA also allowed me to immerse myself in the vibrant culinary scene of the city. I explored new flavors, cuisines, and culinary techniques, constantly seeking to improve my craft as a chef. It was exhilarating to be in a place where creativity and innovation were celebrated, and I embraced the opportunity to experiment with food in exciting and unconventional ways. I found myself captivated by the city's energy and its unique blend of cultures and cuisines.

Living in LA also offered me a chance to collaborate with other experts in the fields of nutrition and fitness. The city was home to a thriving community of health-conscious individuals, and I had the privilege of working alongside some of the brightest minds in the industry. Together, we exchanged knowledge and ideas, constantly pushing the boundaries of what we could achieve in the realm of health and wellness.

But the move to LA was not just about business and career growth; it was also a journey of personal growth and self-discovery. Living in a city that embraced diversity and individuality, I found myself embracing my own uniqueness and confidently pursuing my passions. The support and encouragement I received from my clients, friends, and fellow professionals fueled my determination to excel in my chosen path.

Looking back on my journey, I realized that every step I took, every decision I made, and every challenge I faced had led me to this point in my life.

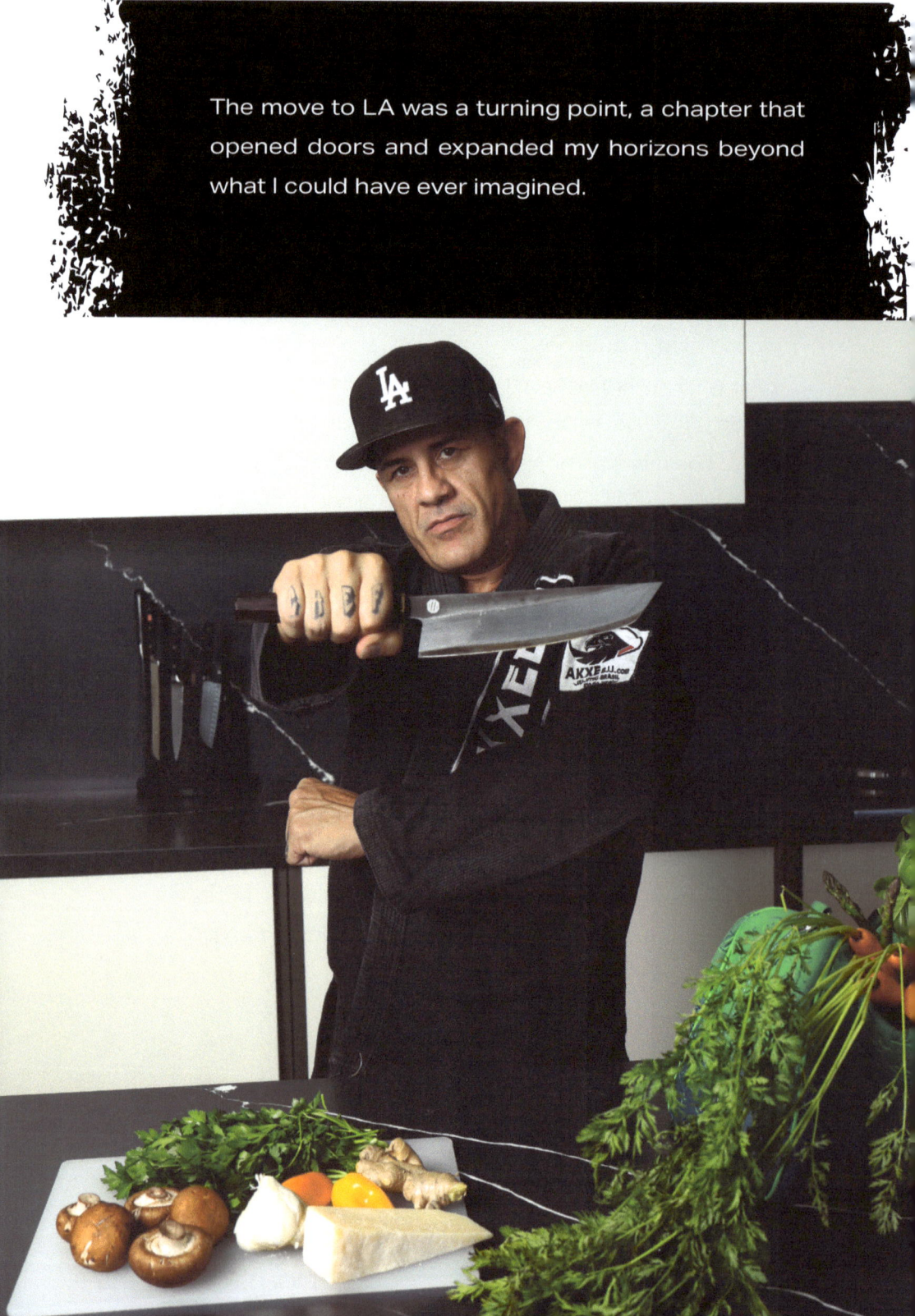

> The move to LA was a turning point, a chapter that opened doors and expanded my horizons beyond what I could have ever imagined.

CHAPTER 7
Healing Through Food with Demi Lovato

As my career blossomed in LA, I had the opportunity to work with some truly remarkable individuals. One of them was the talented Demi Lovato. The chance to collaborate with Demi came through a connection with a company that was in touch with her team. They saw potential in my approach to food and cooking, which they believed could align with Demi's needs and desires. I was excited about the prospect of helping her, knowing that she had struggled with issues related to food, including binge eating and a negative relationship with eating.

Having grown up close to someone who battled bulimia, I understood firsthand the devastating impact that eating disorders could have on a person's physical and mental well-being. I felt that my experiences had prepared me to be a good fit for Demi and her team, and they agreed. I eagerly embraced the opportunity to support her.

My initial meetings were with Demi's team, and it wasn't until later that I had the chance to meet her in person. When we first connected, I spent my days with her. As she and I spent time together, I prepared fresh and wholesome meals, aiming to shift her focus away from processed sugars and foods.

One of the biggest challenges was helping Demi cope with binge eating episodes. We worked together to create a plan that encouraged her to choose natural and earth-grown foods, steering clear of the processed and refined alternatives. It was essential for her to realize that she could enjoy flavorsome treats without compromising her health.

Working closely with her team, especially with a gentleman named Dan, who was very close to Demi, we created a supportive environment for her. I understood the importance of having genuine support around her, as opposed to just "yes" people. Dan and I constantly collaborated to ensure Demi had the best guidance and care.

One of the signature desserts I prepared for Demi was an avocado cheesecake with a quinoa and chia seed crust. I wanted to offer her a treat that she could indulge in without guilt. The dessert was designed to be satisfying yet made with wholesome ingredients that would nourish her body and mind.

I once prepared the avocado cheesecake for a family gathering at Demi's place. Her mother and sisters were present, and I served the dessert with a sprinkle of the crust on top and adorned it with flowers. The response was overwhelmingly positive, and Demi and her family loved the creation. From then on, the avocado cheesecake became a favorite for Demi, and she would often request it.

Witnessing the positive impact of my culinary creations on both Demi's physical and mental health was immensely gratifying. The journey with her was filled with challenges and triumphs, but I knew that every step we took was crucial in her path to healing. The experience further solidified my belief in the powerful connection between food and mental health, and I continued to explore ways to support my clients in their holistic well-being.

As Demi and I worked together, I was inspired to further develop my understanding of food's impact on the body and mind. My studies under Rob Wolf and my passion for exploring scientific research contributed to shaping my own approach to nutrition. I emphasized the importance of natural, earth-grown, and grass-fed ingredients, believing that such foods hold the key to optimal performance.

My work with Demi Lovato was a testament to the transformative impact that food can have on a person's life. I found a sense of purpose and fulfillment in guiding others towards a healthier and happier life through the power of food, but I knew that my mission was far from over. The journey ahead was brimming with opportunities to make a positive difference in the lives of many more individuals, and I was eager to embrace each challenge that lay ahead, armed with the belief that food has the power to heal, nourish, and uplift us on our path to wellness.

CHEF'S TIP

There are a multitude of eating disorders, so it's important to know what you are dealing with before attempting to help through nutrition. People with eating disorders can't do calorie counting because they feel restricted. I use guidelines, rather than a strict calorie count, so people don't feel trapped into a certain way of eating — that way they don't get triggered. People with eating disorders need flexibility, not boundaries.

For example, when working with binge eating, it was important that there was a flexibility to what I was preparing each day. I noticed that with Demi, it helped if I would make similar foods to what she would gravitate towards when she was wanting to binge. For example, she would binge on things like cheesecake, so we made the avocado cheesecake to fill her cheesecake craving in a healthy way. That would also allow her to mentally feel good about it when she was eating.

If you are cooking or meal prepping for someone who has an eating disorder, make sure they are also seeking professional help with their situation from a mental health professional.

For more information, visit
www.nationaleatingdisorders.org.

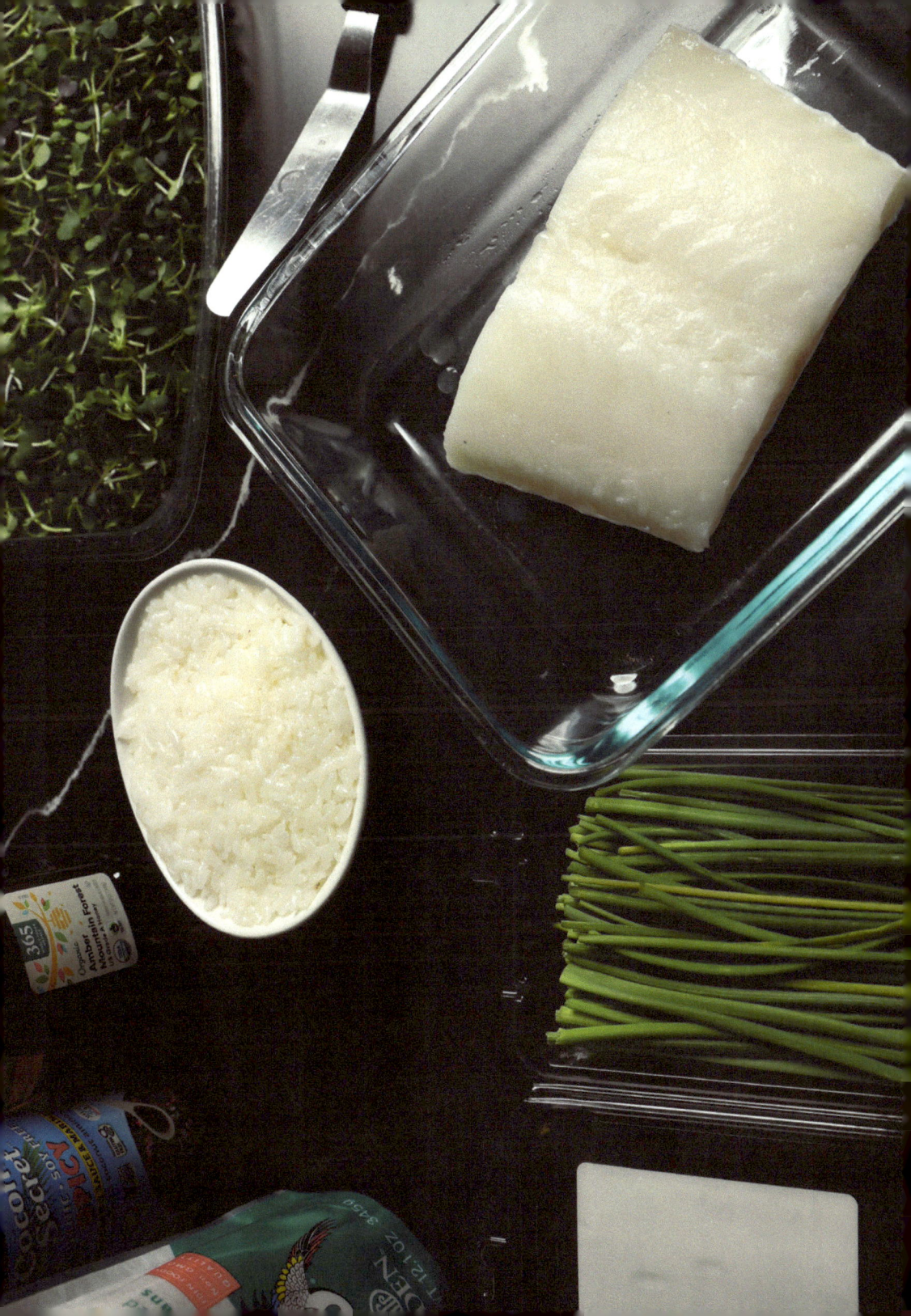

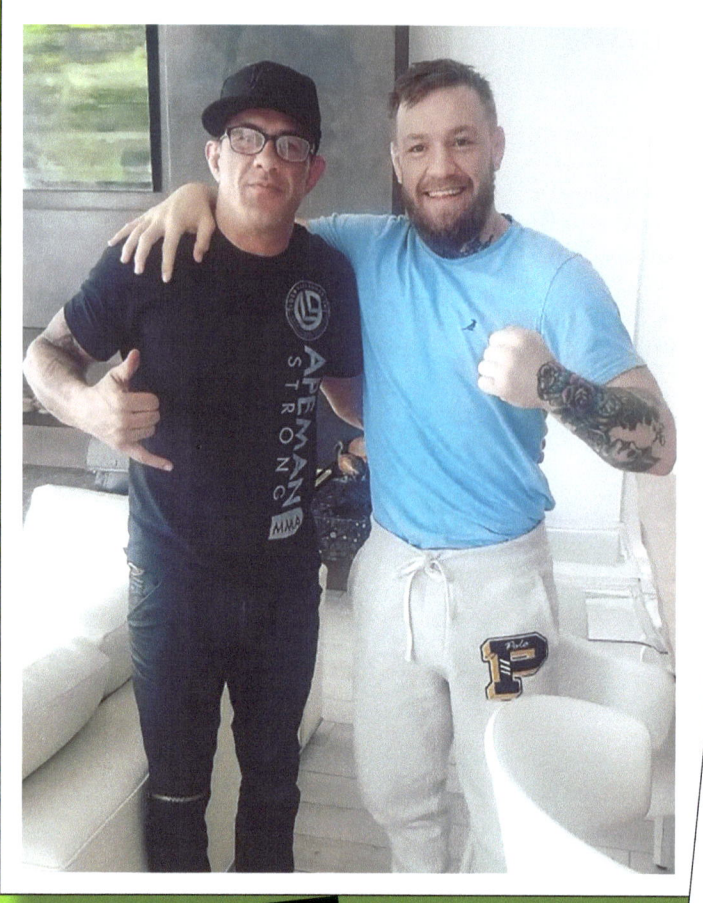
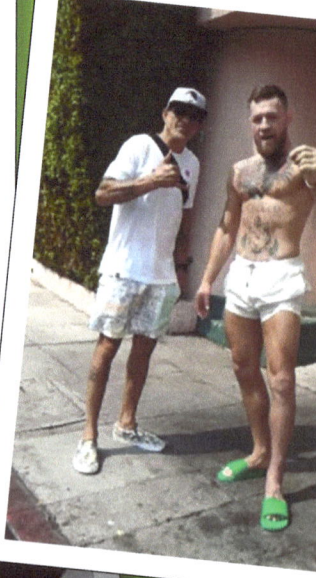

CONOR MCGREGOR

CHAPTER 8

The World of Champions — McGregor vs. Khabib

After my time working with Demi Lovato, my journey took an exhilarating turn as I partnered with a company that specialized in certifying individuals for weight cuts and fighter nutrition. The next phase of my career involved conducting seminars and workshops, not just in the United States, but also in various international locations. From Ireland to London to Florida, I traveled far and wide, sharing my culinary expertise and passion for nutrition with eager learners.

These seminars were a life-changing experience, not only for the participants but also for me. Traveling to new countries and exploring different cultures always brought a sense of wonder and excitement. Moreover, meeting aspiring young individuals who admired my work and looked up to me as a chef and nutritionist was incredibly gratifying. The connections I made during these events turned into lasting friendships, some of which led to collaborations and valuable contributions to my future endeavors.

One such individual, a talented and enthusiastic

man named Dylan Donington, stood out among the attendees. We formed a strong bond, and he became more than just an apprentice; he became a trusted partner in my culinary ventures. Dylan accompanied me to various fight camps, including one that involved the rising boxing sensation, Ryan Garcia. Together, we learned from each other, fine-tuned our skills, and shared our knowledge with the athletes we supported.

Amidst conducting seminars and working with a plethora of UFC fighters, the next significant milestone in my career emerged: the opportunity to be part of a camp with none other than Conor McGregor, ahead of his monumental fight against Khabib Nurmagomedov. The camp took place in the vibrant city of Las Vegas, and it marked a turning point in my culinary journey.

From the moment I met Conor, I recognized that the media's portrayal of him barely scratched the surface of his true character. Beneath the sensational headlines, he proved to be deeply dedicated to his craft and fiercely protective of his team. Working with Conor was a privilege, and it reinforced my understanding of the profound connection between nutrition, discipline, and athletic performance.

Throughout the camp, Conor's commitment and determination were unparalleled. He entrusted me with the crucial task of providing him with the perfect nutrition to fuel his training. Ensuring that he had the optimal sustenance to perform at his peak was a responsibility I approached with utmost care and professionalism. Together, we fine-tuned his meals, making sure they were perfectly balanced to enhance his training and recovery.

The experience of working with Conor was truly transformative, deepening my appreciation for the culinary arts and nutrition's pivotal role in the world of champions. The trust placed in me by Conor and his team was a testament to the expertise I had honed over the years. The camp not only solidified our professional relationship but also left a lasting impact on my career, opening doors to new opportunities and pushing me to strive for excellence in every culinary creation.

My career trajectory now involved working with a multitude of fighters, including renowned athletes like Daniel Cormier and Israel Adesanya. Each fight camp presented unique challenges, but I thrived in the fast-paced and high-pressure environment. Guiding fighters through their nutritional needs and witnessing their progress towards victory filled me with immense satisfaction.

Beyond the octagon, I continued my mission of educating others about proper nutrition and culinary arts. Conducting seminars and workshops remained an integral part of my life as I aimed to inspire and empower the next generation of chefs and nutritionists. The joy of sharing my knowledge and expertise with eager learners was immeasurable.

As the curtain rose on each new chapter of my career, I embraced the ever-changing landscape with enthusiasm and dedication. The world of champions had become my home, and I was determined to leave a mark with every culinary creation, every nutrition plan, and every fighter I supported.

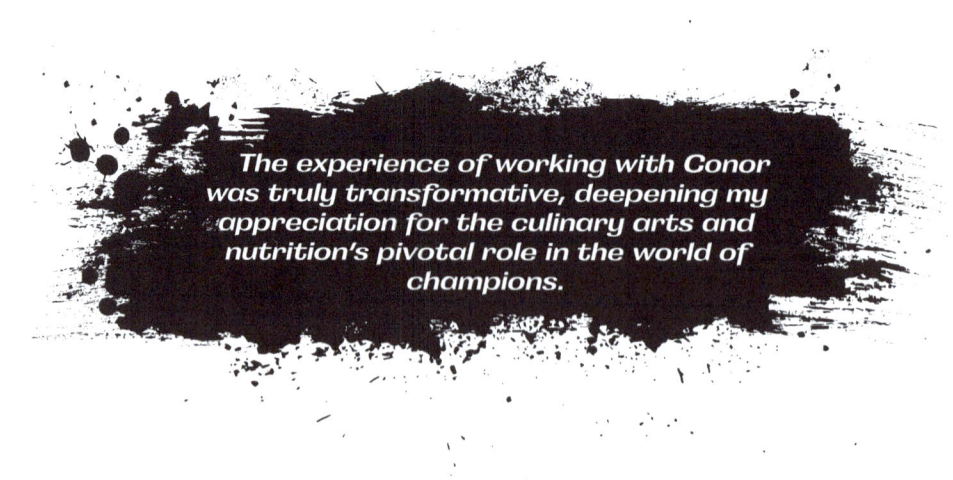

The experience of working with Conor was truly transformative, deepening my appreciation for the culinary arts and nutrition's pivotal role in the world of champions.

CHAPTER 9

A Culinary Knockout — KSI and the Black Cod Revelation

As my culinary journey continued, a new and exciting opportunity knocked on my door — working with KSI, the renowned YouTuber-turned-boxer. The path that led me to KSI was a result of my association with a company that connected me with fighters and influencers, and they recommended me to KSI's team for his upcoming rematch with Logan Paul.

From the first meeting, I knew this collaboration was destined to be a success. Our energies aligned seamlessly, and I found KSI to be an easy-going and down-to-earth personality. His determination to excel in the boxing world complemented my straightforward and blunt approach to nutrition, creating the perfect synergy for our partnership.

As we embarked on this journey, we set our sights on Las Vegas, where the majority of KSI's training camp took place at a rented Airbnb. My role as his nutritionist and chef was to ensure that he received the ideal meals, snacks, and supplements to support his training and overall well-being. To monitor his sleep and energy levels, I used various tools, such as Fitbit or Apple Watch, in addition to

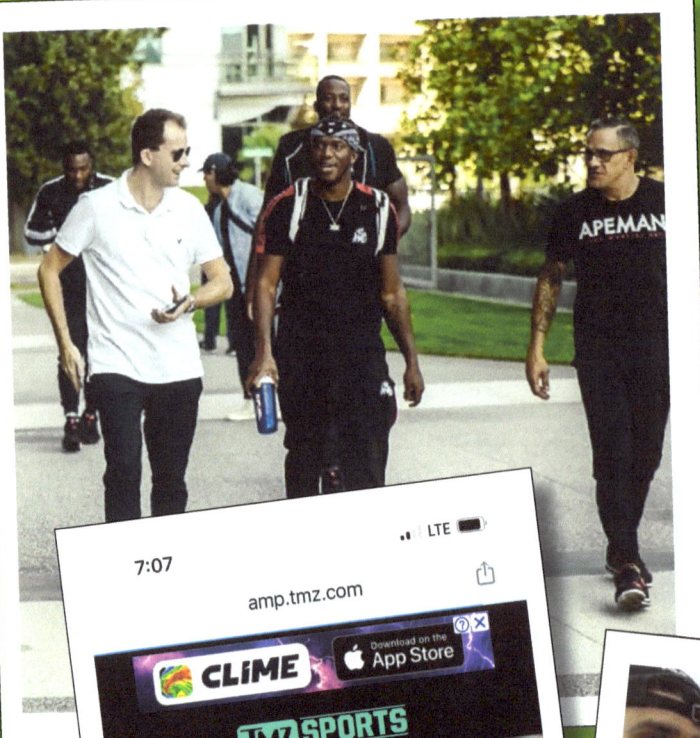
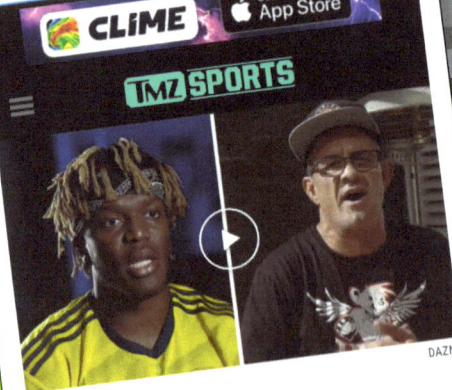

regular conversations to stay attuned to his body's needs.

Understanding the significance of quality sleep in athletic performance, I stressed the importance of proper rest, highlighting that it was during sleep when the body healed, restored, and rejuvenated. My goal was to optimize KSI's potential for the rigorous training ahead and maximize his chances of victory in the upcoming fight.

KSI's transition from a YouTube sensation to a boxer was groundbreaking, and he was among the first to venture into this new arena with such

> To ensure that I could offer the best support the fighters, I meticulously gathered information from each of them, including their preferences, dislikes, allergies, and dietary restrictions.

a massive fan following. With over 20 million subscribers on his YouTube channel, KSI had already demonstrated his charisma and talent as an entertainer before stepping into the boxing ring.

The rematch against Logan Paul was a highly anticipated event, and I was thrilled to be part of KSI's preparation. Throughout the training camp,

KSI demonstrated his commitment and dedication, diligently following the nutrition plan and training regimen laid out for him. As the fight day drew closer, excitement filled the air, and the Coliseum in Los Angeles hosted a sold-out event, setting the stage for an epic showdown.

The fight itself was a nail-biting spectacle, with both fighters displaying their hunger for victory. KSI and Logan Paul fought fiercely, giving their all in every round. It was an evenly matched contest, and the decision eventually went in favor of KSI, marking a moment of triumph in his boxing career.

Reflecting on the experience of working with KSI, there was not one singular standout moment. Instead, it was the entire journey that left an impression on me. Witnessing his dedication, the camaraderie among his team, and the thrill of victory created memories that would be cherished for a lifetime.

Throughout the training camp, I had the chance to connect with KSI on a personal level, discovering his favorite dishes and flavors. One such dish was the black cod from Nobu, a renowned restaurant. Eager to give him a taste of his favorite dish while adhering to my principles of using organic and unprocessed ingredients, I crafted a modified version of the dish. Replacing white sugar with local raw honey and using fermented black miso, I presented KSI with a nourishing and delicious rendition of his beloved meal.

KSI's reaction to the black cod was priceless. The moment he entered the room, the aroma greeted him, and he immediately recognized the dish he adored. His heartfelt appreciation and excitement filled the air, and I knew I had hit the mark in satisfying his taste buds while keeping his nutritional needs in mind.

Beyond my work with KSI, I continued to educate others on the importance of gut health and the microbiome. Staying hydrated, avoiding processed foods, incorporating fermented foods like kimchi or sauerkraut, and consuming natural digestive aids like papaya were key tips I shared with individuals looking to maintain a healthy gut.

The experience of working with KSI was yet another stepping stone in my culinary journey, instilling in me a profound sense of fulfillment and accomplishment. As I eagerly embraced every new opportunity that came my way, I knew that my dedication to the craft, paired with my genuine care for the well-being of my clients, would continue to fuel my success as a nutritionist and chef in the world of champions.

CHAPTER 10

Working with Logan Paul

While at a press conference for the KSI vs. Logan Paul rematch, I remember catching the curious gaze of Logan's manager, Jeff. This moment sparked the possibility of collaborating with Logan in the future.

Several months later, I received an exciting call from Logan's team, inviting me to join his boxing camp as he prepared to face Floyd Mayweather. With enthusiasm, I embarked on this journey, eager to work closely with Logan, a fighter I had previously met and admired.

From the very start, I was by Logan's side every day, ensuring he had the right nutrition to support his intense training sessions. We spent hours together, discussing his goals and fine-tuning his meals to cater to his unique tastes and preferences. Logan's authenticity and generosity made me feel valued and cared for during our time together.

Preparing for the Mayweather fight was a challenging journey with the bout date continuously being pushed back. Our camp extended for months, but Logan's determination never faltered. We trained diligently in Puerto Rico, perfecting his skills and staying ready for the eventual face-off in Miami.

Logan's down-to-earth nature stood out as he treated everyone around him like family. His warmth and kindness made the training environment enjoyable for all of us. His love for simple comfort food, particularly butter noodles, held a special place in his heart as it reminded him of his mom's cooking from his childhood. I made sure to recreate this dish in a healthier way, using raw Parmesan cheese and grass-fed butter, aligning it with his training diet.

Beyond the boxing preparations, our bond went beyond a professional relationship. Logan's infectious enthusiasm brightened each day, and we shared stories, laughter, and learned from one another, forming a genuine friendship.

Throughout the extended wait for the fight, Logan's unwavering determination was admirable. We faced challenges together, adapting to the ever-changing circumstances, and he maintained his focus and motivation to showcase his skills in the ring.

When the momentous fight in Miami finally arrived, excitement filled the air. Logan faced Floyd Mayweather, a legendary boxer, and although the outcome wasn't a traditional victory, he achieved something extraordinary by going toe-to-toe with Mayweather.

Our journey extended beyond the boxing match. Logan's generosity and thoughtfulness made a lasting impact on me. He treated me to unforgettable experiences, such as private jet trips and exquisite dinners, making me feel like a valued member of his team. Our connection went beyond the professional realm, blossoming into a genuine friendship.

Working with Logan was truly life-changing. His passion for his craft, combined with his kindness and authenticity, left a profound impression on me. He proved to be not just a social media influencer but a dedicated athlete, and I was honored to be a part of his journey.

As we concluded the camp, I felt grateful for the privilege of working with exceptional individuals like KSI and Logan Paul. In the end, it wasn't just about the fights or the fame. It was about the connections, the lessons, and the friendships that enriched my life as a nutritionist and chef. My path had led me to work with some of the most prominent names in the industry, and I was grateful for every moment of it. The lessons I learned from these remarkable fighters shaped my career and inspired me to continue making a positive impact in the world of champions.

CHAPTER 11
From Injury to Recovery with Conor McGregor

After my unforgettable experience working with Logan Paul, I was presented with a new opportunity — to be part of Conor McGregor's team for his fight against Dustin Poirier. I found myself back at side of one of the biggest names in the world of combat sports.

Leaving behind the excitement of the Logan Paul camp, I joined Conor's team with a renewed sense of enthusiasm. Our preparations took us to Orange County, away from the hustle and bustle of Las Vegas. It was a more intimate setting, with Conor, his trusted trainer, Tristan, and the rest of the team focused on the upcoming battle.

Days turned into weeks, and our bond grew stronger as we trained, laughed, and shared moments of camaraderie. The calm and peaceful environment allowed us to focus on honing Conor's skills and preparing him mentally and physically for the fight.

Finally, the day of the bout arrived, and the energy was electric. Conor's unwavering determination was palpable as he stepped into the ring with Dustin

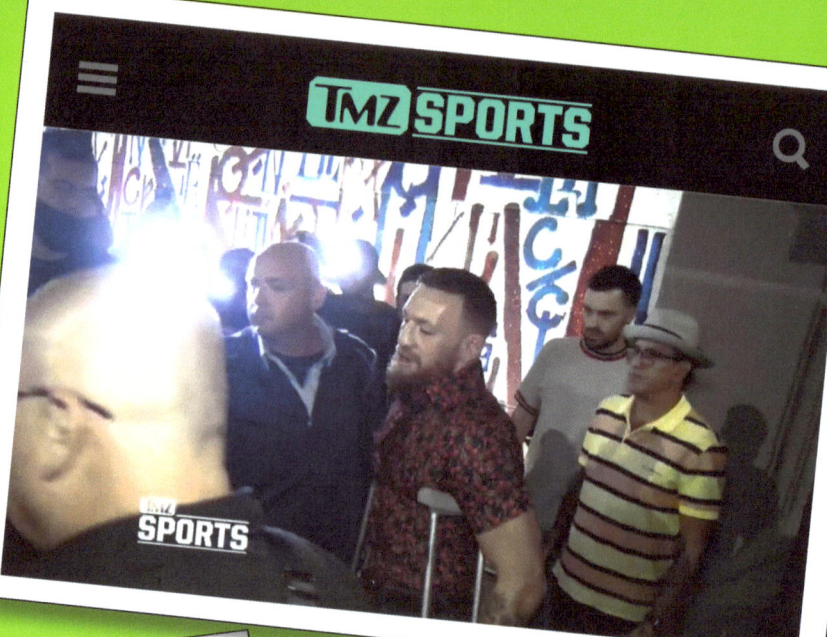

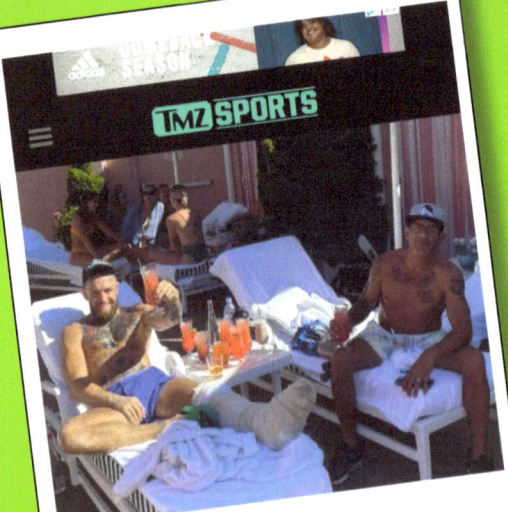

BREAKING NEWS

CONOR MCGREGOR
RECOVERING POOLSIDE IN L.A.
... All Smiles 1 Week After Surgery

7/22/2021 6:17 AM PT

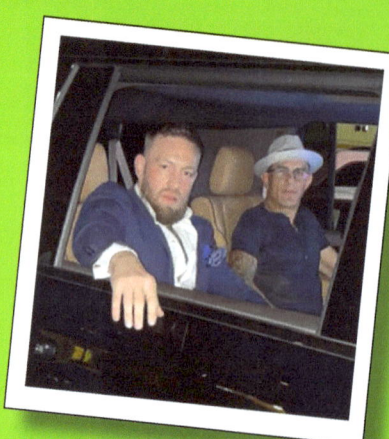

Poirier. However, fate had different plans, and Conor suffered a devastating leg injury during the fight. It was a challenging moment for all of us, but we rallied together to support Conor during his immediate recovery.

In the days following the fight, I stayed by Conor's side, ensuring he received the best possible care. Alongside his medical team, we worked tirelessly to provide him with the nutrition and support he needed to begin his healing process.

As Conor's recovery progressed, we traveled from LA to Miami, and then to Italy, Ireland, and finally to Dubai. Each step of the journey was marked with Conor's determination and resilience. His commitment to getting back in shape and regaining his strength was awe-inspiring.

Witnessing Conor's unwavering dedication during those months was a life-changing experience for me. He demonstrated not only the mindset of a champion but also the heart of a fighter who would never back down from a challenge.

Through the ups and downs of his healing journey, Conor showed incredible character and spirit. He faced setbacks with courage, and each day, he pushed himself to new limits, proving that he was more than just a fighter — he was a true warrior.

As the months passed, Conor's hard work and dedication paid off, and he made his triumphant return to the ring. The journey from injury to recovery was a testament to his indomitable spirit and the unyielding support of his team.

Being a part of Conor McGregor's healing journey was an honor and a privilege. It taught me the importance of perseverance, teamwork, and never losing sight of one's goals. Conor's journey will forever inspire me in my own culinary and nutritional endeavors.

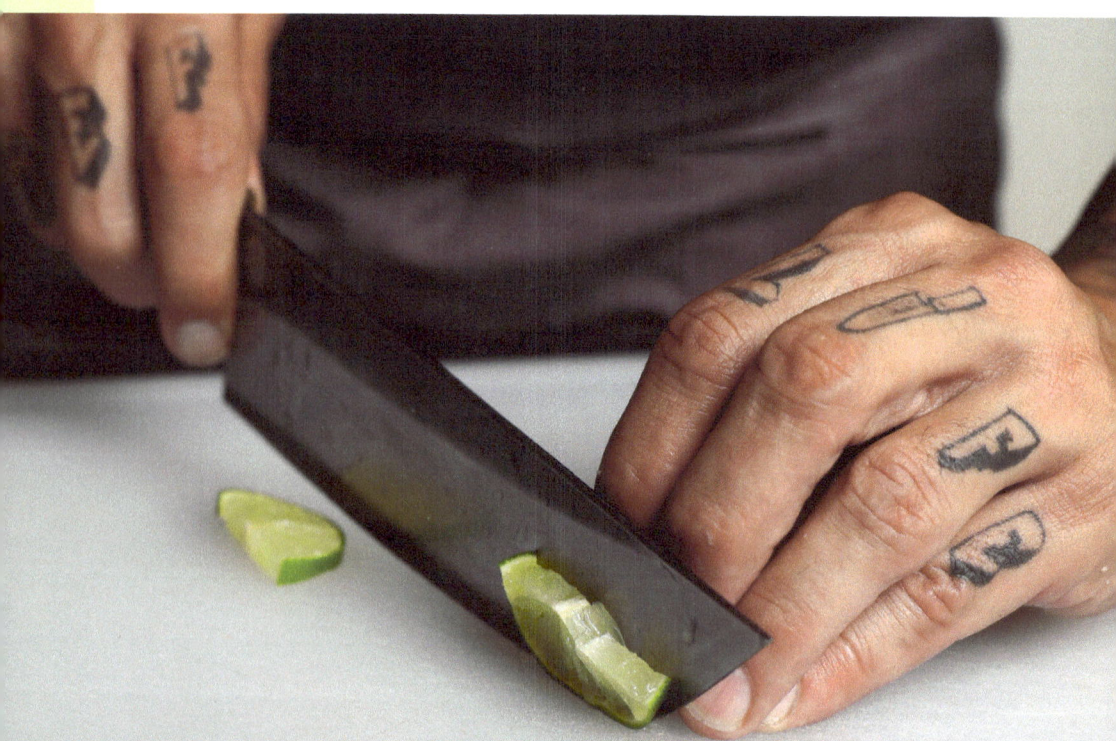

CHAPTER 12

Embracing New Challenges — Working with Influencer Boxers

After concluding my time with Conor McGregor, I returned to Los Angeles, taking some time off to rest and reflect on my next steps. After settling back in, I soon received a call from Logan Paul, beckoning me back to Puerto Rico to continue our collaboration.

For the next seven months, I resided in Puerto Rico, assuming the role of a full-time chef and nutritionist for Logan. My primary focus was to ensure he maintained a healthy lifestyle, supporting him during his WWE endeavors. This rigorous form of entertainment demanded careful weight management and proper nutrition to keep him at peak performance levels.

Though there were no fight camps during this period, my responsibilities were vital in keeping Logan ready for potential future fights. Moreover, it was a period of growth and exploration for both of us, as Logan's influence as a social media personality opened doors to working with crossover boxers and influencers in the world of combat sports.

As I transitioned from working with professional fighters to influencers and YouTubers, I found myself preparing for the exciting new domain of crossover boxing. Among the influencers I collaborated with were individuals like Tayler Holder, who had trained with renowned boxers like Canelo and Ryan Garcia.

One of the highlights of this phase was my involvement in a fight camp with a promising crossover boxer named Dakota Miller. His drive and ambition left a lasting impression on me as we worked together to prepare him for his moment in the ring.

The shift in my career allowed me to explore this emerging space of crossover boxing, where influencers and YouTubers ventured into the world of professional fighting. Working with these individuals provided a fresh perspective, presenting its own unique set of challenges and opportunities.

Among the promotions I started working with was KSI's misfits, where I collaborated with several fighters and boxers. The atmosphere was different from the high-stress, high-pressure events I had experienced previously, but it offered its own set of rewards.

In this new chapter, I also continued my journey with Logan Paul, who had a forthcoming fight on the horizon. Despite the events being less publicized, the experiences were no less valuable, and the relationships I formed with these individuals were just as meaningful.

This phase in my career allowed me to take a step back from the intensity of high-level events, providing a breathing space to focus on other aspects of my life and career. I embraced the opportunity to develop and foster other parts of my culinary journey, seeking out new challenges and avenues for growth.

As I look back on my culinary odyssey, I am grateful for the diverse range of individuals I have had the privilege to work with. Each chapter has enriched my expertise and shaped my approach as a nutritionist and chef. From working with celebrated fighters to collaborating with influencers and crossover boxers, every experience has left an indelible mark on my journey.

The road ahead is filled with endless possibilities, and I am eager to continue making a positive impact on the lives of those I encounter, regardless of their background or level of prominence. Through culinary excellence and nutrition guidance, I strive to fuel the success of champions, inspiring them to achieve greatness inside and outside the ring.

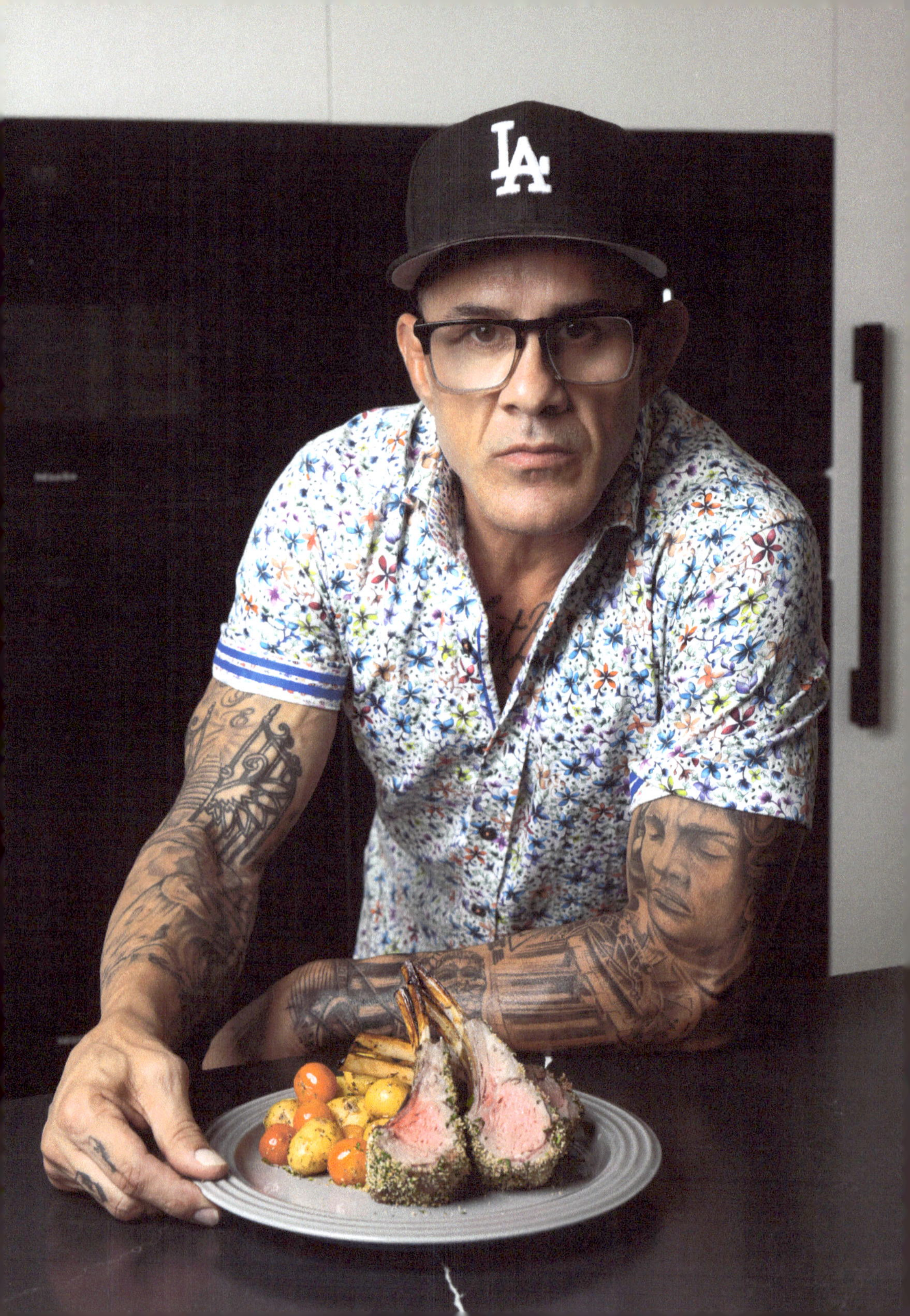

THE FOOD

ITEMS I RECOMMEND FOR THE KITCHEN

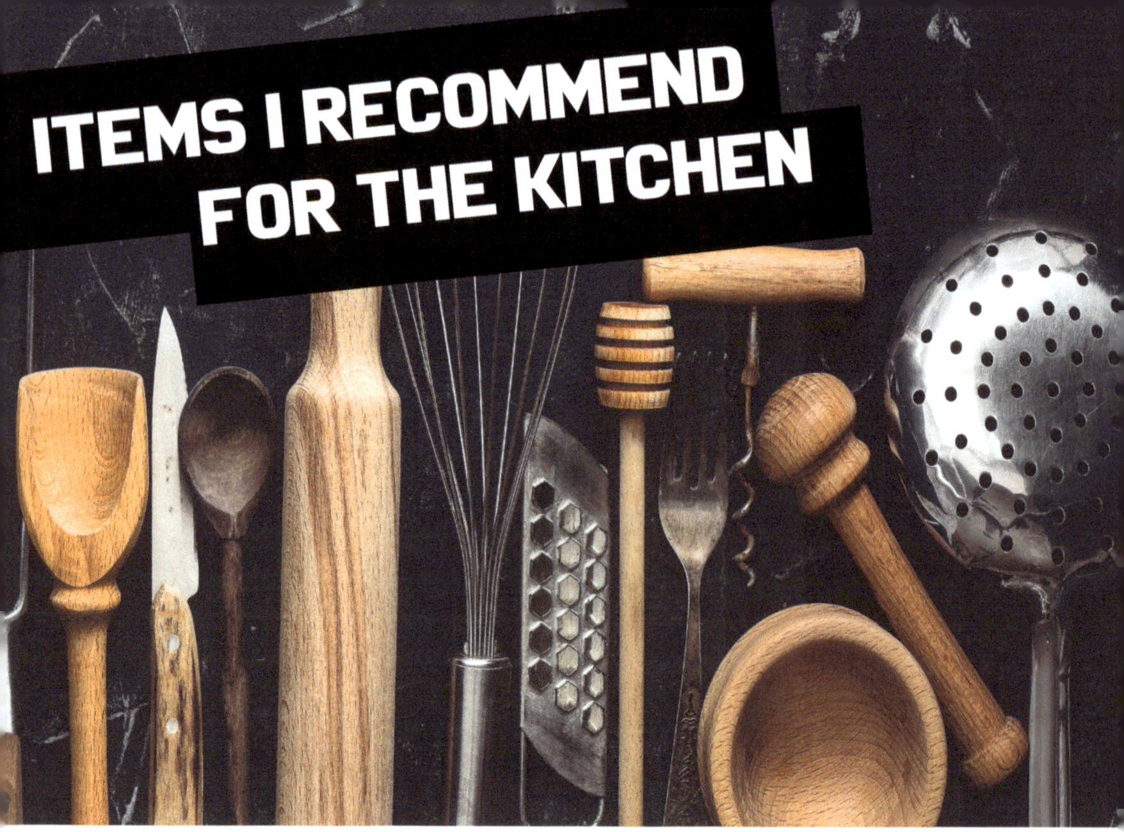

- Spatula
- Measuring Spoons
- Measuring Cups
- Food Scale
- Blender
- Food Processor
- Cast Iron Skillet
- Sharp Knives
- Food Scale
- Protein Thermometer

With this book, you are going to find recipes that require many different ingredients. What I like to do, whether cooking for myself or for a client, is make sure that I am getting the best ingredients available in that area. I put a lot of effort into ensuring that the meals I cook are clean.

My recommendation for you to would be to source out local farmers markets. Use all organic ingredients as much as possible. Use grass-fed, grass finished beef, free range chickens and eggs, and use fresh caught fish rather than farm raised.

Having a healthy diet doesn't start with what you're putting into your body; it goes back to where that food came from as well, what was put into any meat you're consuming, and what was added to any crop. It goes back to the old adage of: You are what you eat. So before you start cooking, make sure that what you're putting into your meals are healthy.

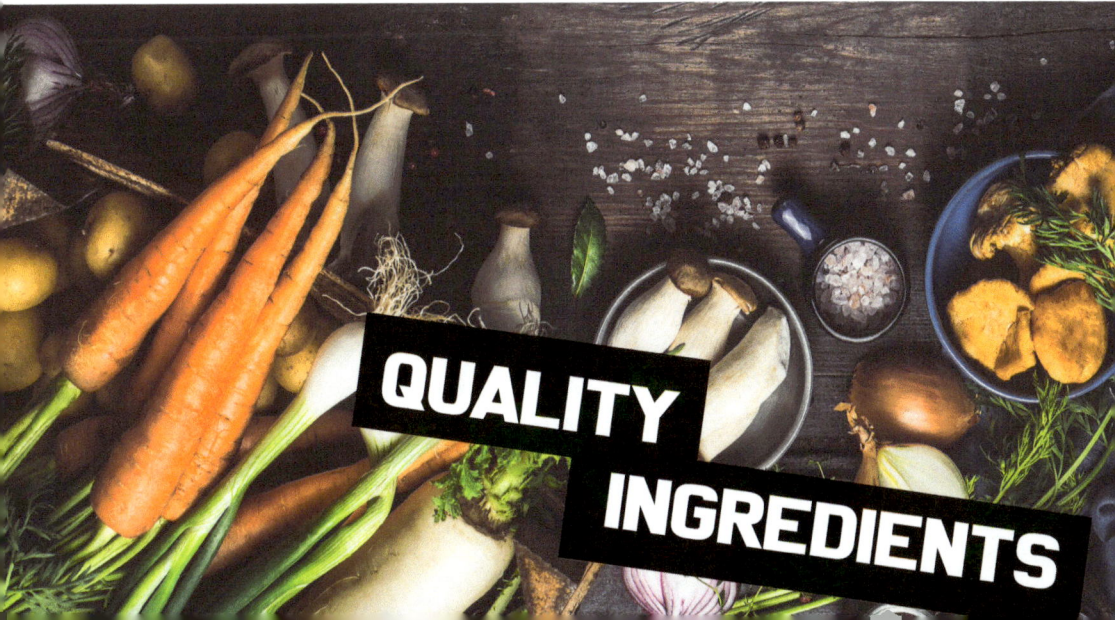

QUALITY INGREDIENTS

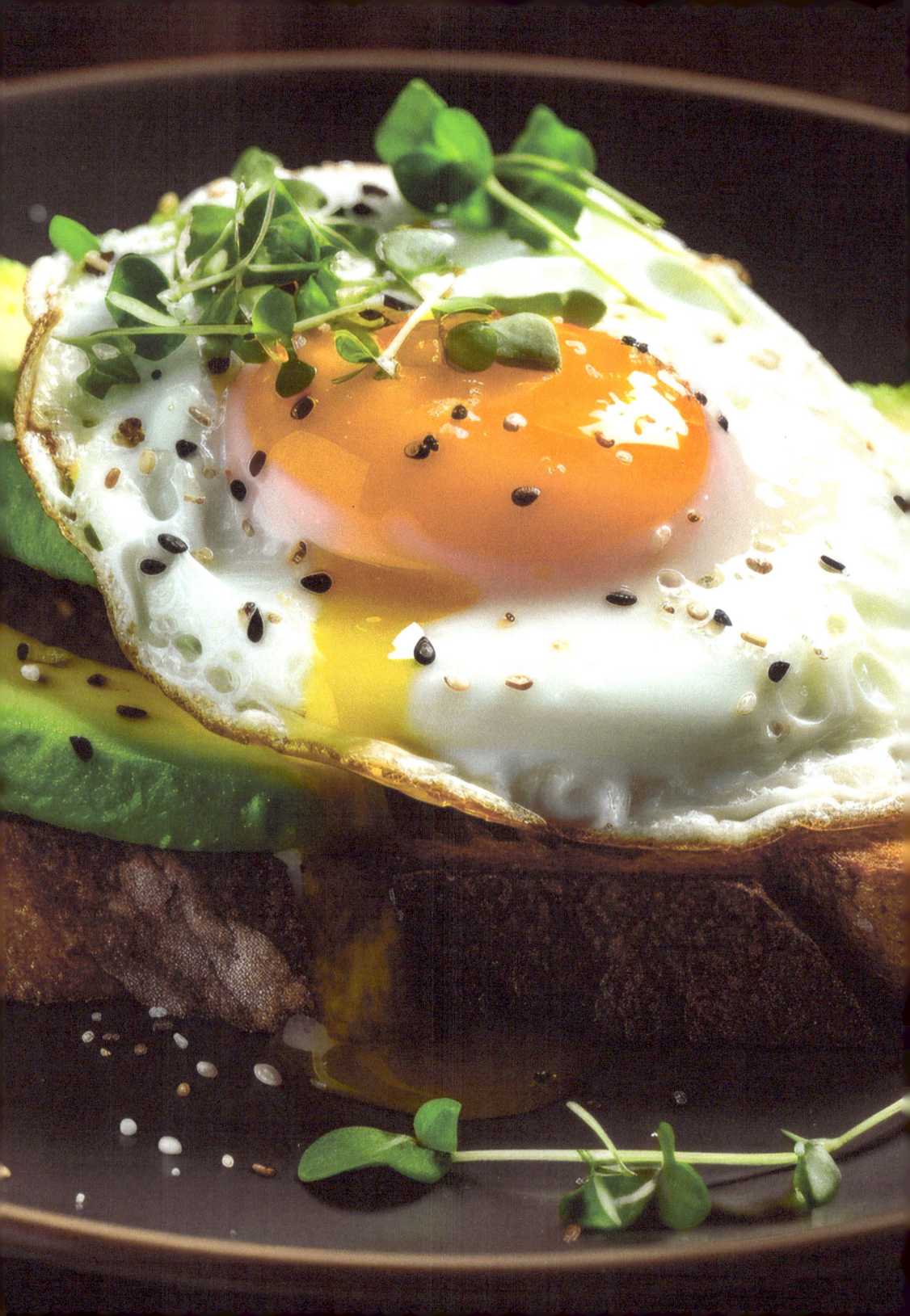

BREAKFAST

EGG, MUSHROOM, AND AVOCADO SCRAMBLE WITH CHICKEN SAUSAGE

INGREDIENTS

- 3 Eggs
- ¼ Cup Mushroom
- ½ Avocado (Chopped)
- 1 Granny Smith Apple, Unpeeled
- 1 lb Ground Chicken
- 2 Garlic Cloves (Finally Minced)
- 2 Scallions (Chopped)
- 1 Tsp Kosher Salt
- ½ Tsp Black Pepper
- ½ Tsp Fennel Seeds
- ¼ Tsp Crushed Red Pepper
- Pinch Of Nutmeg
- 4 Tsp Olive Oil (Divided)

PREPARING THE DISH

EGGS

1. Put a skillet on medium heat and melt a little grass fed butter inside. Throw in mushrooms, add a pinch of salt, and sauté for a few minutes. When mushrooms are down, drain the liquid and wipe out pan. Put back on medium heat. Scramble eggs and season with a little salt, pepper, and garlic powder to taste. Pour eggs into the pan along with mushrooms. Use a rubber spatula to push eggs from the outside of the pan in towards the middle. Continue to do this until eggs are the consistency that you like. Toss in the avocado right when eggs are done and lightly mix together.

SAUSAGE

2. Grate the apple on the large holes of a box grater onto a cutting board; discard the core and stem. Put the grated apple on a paper towel and carefully wring out the juice while reserving the apple. Roughly chop the grated apple and put into a large bowl.

3. Add the ground chicken, garlic, scallions, salt, pepper, fennel seeds, crushed red pepper, and nutmeg to the bowl with the apple. Using your hands, mix all ingredients together. Shape into 8 balls and place on a parchment-lined baking sheet.

4. Heat 2 teaspoons of the oil in a large cast iron skillet over medium heat. Flatten the balls, each into a 3-inch-wide patties, and place in the preheated skillet. Cook the sausage patties until browned on both sides and cooked through, 6 to 8 minutes. When done, serve alongside eggs, omelets, or whatever you desire.

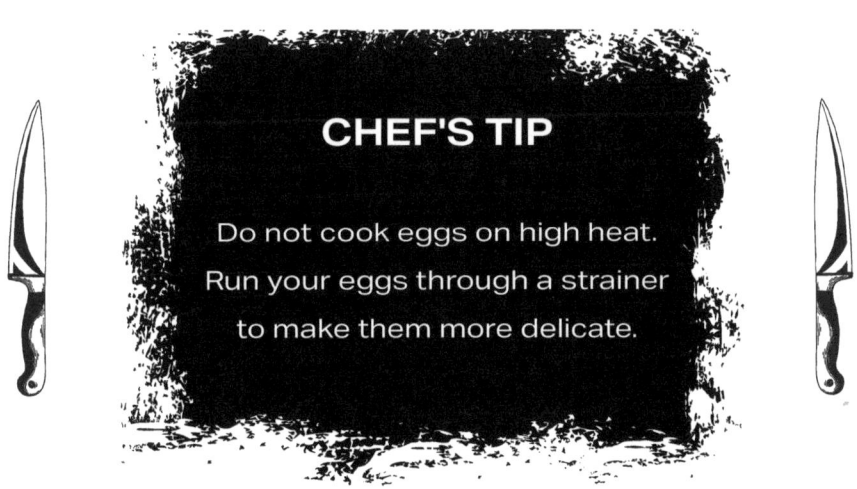

CHEF'S TIP

Do not cook eggs on high heat. Run your eggs through a strainer to make them more delicate.

POTATO, ONION, AND ZUCCHINI FRITTATA

INGREDIENTS

- 1 Small Russet Potato (Peeled and Cut Into 1/2-Inch Cubes)
- 4 Large Eggs
- 2 Egg Whites
- 2 Tbsp Coarsely Chopped Fresh Cilantro Leaves
- ¾ Tsp Salt
- ¼ Tsp Red Chili Flakes (Optional)
- 1 Tbsp Olive Oil
- 1 Garlic Clove (Minced)
- 1 Small Onion (Finely Chopped)
- 1 Small Zucchini, About. 6 Oz (Grated and Squeezed Dry)
- ½ Cup Goat Cheese (2–3 Oz)
- 2 Strips of Turkey Bacon (Cooked And Thinly Sliced) (Optional)

PREPARING THE DISH

1. Put a medium-sized pot over medium heat and cook the potatoes until tender (about 8 min).
2. In a large bowl, whisk together the eggs, egg whites, cilantro, salt, and red chili flakes.
3. Preheat the oven broiler to medium-high.
4. In a 10-inch, oven-safe, nonstick skillet, heat the oil over medium-high heat. Add the garlic and onion and cook, stirring occasionally, until the onion is translucent (2 min). Add zucchini and cook until tender (about 6 minutes).
5. Add the cooked potatoes and cook, stirring occasionally. When the potatoes start to brown (about 3–4 min), evenly pour the egg mixture over the vegetables. Cook over medium heat. Tilt the pan and lift the edges of the mixture with a rubber spatula to let the uncooked egg flow

underneath. Crumble up the goat cheese and add it along with the turkey bacon. Broil 7 inches from the heat until the eggs rise slightly and are set. The cheese should be golden brown (about 5 minutes). Let cool on the countertop for 5 minutes, then cut and serve.

EVERYTHING BAGEL CRUSTED SALMON OVER ARUGULA SALAD

INGREDIENTS

- 2 6-Oz Skin-On Salmon Fillets
- Pink Himalayan Salt
- Freshly Ground Black Pepper
- 2 Tbsp Spicy Harissa Paste
- 3 Tbsp Everything Bagel Seasoning
- 3 Tbsp Extra-Virgin Olive Oil, Divided
- 1 ½ Oz Cream Cheese (About 3 Tbsp), Softened
- 1 Small Shallot (Finely Chopped), Divided
- ¼ Fresh Dill (Chopped), Divided
- 2 Tbsp Fresh Lemon Juice (Divided In Half)
- 2 Oz Arugula
- 6 Oz Cherry Tomatoes (Halved)
- 1 Mini Cucumber (Cut Into ¼"-Thick Rounds)
- 1 Tbsp Drained Capers (Coarsely Chopped)

PREPARING THE DISH

1. Preheat oven to 425°.
2. Place a large cast-iron skillet in the oven.
3. Pat salmon dry, then season all over with 1 teaspoon salt and a pinch of pepper. Spread harissa onto salmon flesh. Sprinkle each fillet with everything bagel seasoning.
4. Carefully remove skillet from oven and drizzle with 2 tablespoons oil. Arrange salmon in skillet, skin side down. Bake until flesh becomes opaque and easily flakes with a fork, about 10 to 12 minutes.
5. Meanwhile, in a small bowl, whisk cream cheese, half of shallot, 1 tablespoon dill, 1 tablespoon lemon juice, 2 tablespoons water, and remaining 1 tablespoon oil until

smooth; season with a pinch of salt. In another small bowl, soak remaining shallots with remaining lemon juice.

6. In a large bowl, toss arugula, tomato, cucumber, capers, marinated shallots, and remaining 3 tablespoons of dill. Add half of dressing and toss. Divide salmon among plates. Serve with salad and remaining dressing.

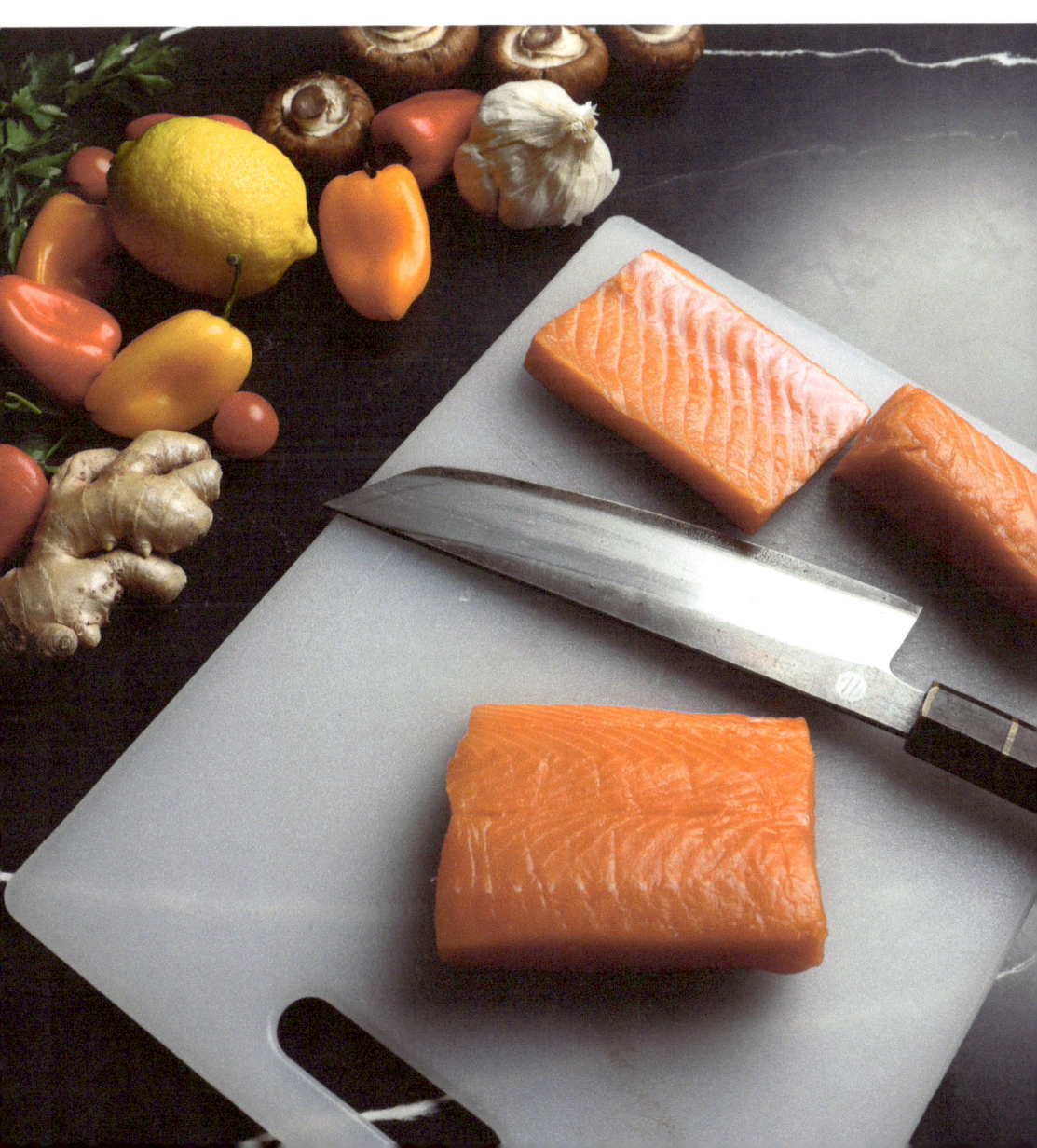

SIMPLE EGG SCRAMBLE WITH BABY POTATOES, BELL PEPPER, AND ONION

INGREDIENTS

- 3 Eggs
- 1 Cup Baby Potatoes (Cut In Half)
- ½ Bell Pepper (Chopped)
- ¼ Cup Onion (Chopped)
- ½ Tomato (Chopped)
- ¼ Tsp Garlic Powder (Or 2 Cloves Chopped Garlic, Finely Minced)
- Salt and Pepper

PREPARING THE DISH

1. Scramble the eggs in a bowl and set aside. Chop up all veggies and potatoes and set aside.
2. Fill a pot half way with water, add a little salt and bring to a boil. Add the potatoes to the water and cook for about 8 min or until soft.
3. While the potatoes are cooking, get a pan and put it on medium heat. Sauté the veggies for about 3 min. Add the potatoes into the pan with the veggies and mix in your eggs. Add a little salt and pepper to taste.

EGG AND GOAT CHEESE SCRAMBLE WITH VEGGIES

INGREDIENTS

- 1 Tbsp Unsalted Butter
- 4 Eggs
- ¼ Cup Milk
- 2 Oz Goat Cheese (Crumbled)
- ½ Cup Bell Pepper (Diced)
- ½ Cup Halved Cherry Tomatoes
- 1 Avocado (Diced)
- Parsley
- Fresh Ground Black Pepper

PREPARING THE DISH

1. Melt butter in a skillet over medium heat. Add the bell pepper and a pinch of little salt and pepper. Cook for 4 to 5 minutes, until softened.

2. While peppers are cooking, mix together eggs, milk, cherry tomatoes, and 1 oz. of goat cheese.

3. Reduce the heat to medium-low and pour the egg mixture into the pan. Let cook for 1–2 minutes, until the eggs begin to set. Once they start to set, push the eggs from the edges to the center of the pan and push them in. Once cooked to your liking, top with remaining goat cheese and cut up avocado.

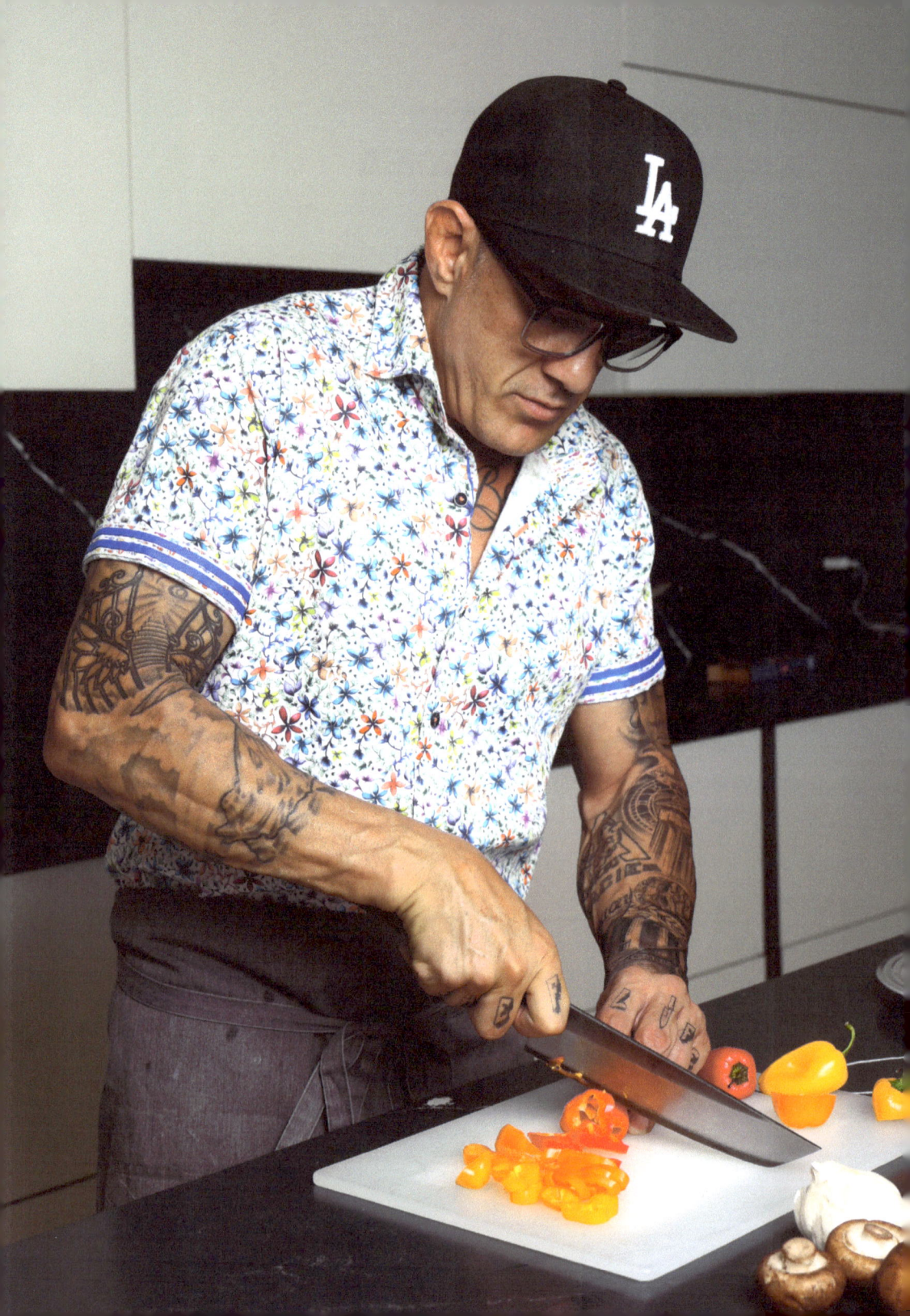

AVOCADO TOAST WITH EGGS, CHERRY TOMATOES, AND SPINACH

INGREDIENTS

- 4 Slices Sprouted Grain Bread (Or Bread of Choice)
- 1 Avocado
- 4 Eggs
- 1 Tbsp Milk
- 1 Tbsp Grass Fed Butter
- 8 Cherry Tomatoes (Halved)
- ½ Cup Spinach
- Salt and Pepper
- Garlic Powder
- Chives (Finely Chopped)

PREPARING THE DISH

1. Toast the bread in the toaster and set aside. Finely mash the avocado while mixing in garlic powder and salt to taste. Spread the mashed avocado over the toast and put it on a plate.

2. Beat the eggs with 1 tablespoon of milk in a mixing bowl and set aside.

3. Preheat a non-stick frying pan on medium head. Add the butter in the pan once heated. Lower the heat slightly and add in the eggs. Toss in the spinach and cook down. When spinach is wilted, add eggs. Cook until the eggs are to your liking. Split the scrambled eggs among the two pieces of toast. Then top with the chopped chives and sliced cherry tomatoes. Crack a little fresh black pepper over the top or more salt if desired.

CRÊPES WITH FRESH FRUIT COMPOTE AND OVER EASY EGGS

INGREDIENTS

- 6 Eggs
- 1 ½ Cups Raw Milk
- 1 Cup Organic Flower
- Pinch Of Salt (Pink Himalayan)
- 1 Tsp Butter
- ½ Cup Blueberries
- ½ Cup Raspberries
- ½ Cup Bananas
- 2 Tbsp Raw Honey
- 3 Tbsp Chapped Walnuts

PREPARING THE DISH

CRÊPES

1. In a bowl, mix together 3 eggs and milk. In a separate bowl, sift flour. (If you do not have a sifter, then whisk the flour for about 60 seconds.) Once flour is sifted, add the milk and egg mixture and whisk together.
2. Heat up a medium-sized skillet to medium heat. Pour a small amount of cold pressed oil or grass fed butter in the pan. Pour 1/4 cup of crepe mixture into pan. Roll the pan to spread the mixture and cook for about 2 min. Flip with a spatula and cook for another minute or until light golden brown.

EGGS

3. Heat up a skillet to medium heat. Add 1 tbsp of butter and let melt. Crack your eggs into the pan and sprinkle with a little salt. Cook eggs until almost all the egg whites are set. Flip the eggs, add a little black pepper, then cook for another 30–40 seconds. You can cook longer if you do not like your yolks runny.

FRUIT COMPOTE

4. Chop up your fruit of choice. When done, place them in a pot on medium heat and add the raw honey. Cook for about 4 min or until it starts to slightly boil. When it comes to a boil, cook for another 2 min, stirring consistently and slowly, to keep the shape of the fruit. Remove from heat. Mix in the chopped nuts, then serve over rolled crêpes.

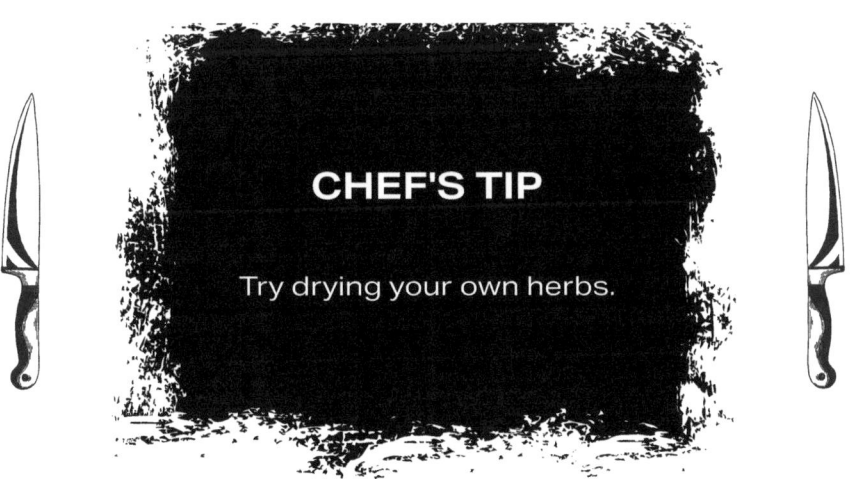

CHEF'S TIP

Try drying your own herbs.

FRIED EGG SANDWICH WITH AVOCADO, SRIRACHA, MAYO, AND MICRO GREENS

INGREDIENTS

- 3 Eggs
- 2 Pieces Sprouted Grain Bread
- 1 Tbsp Sriracha
- ¼ Avocado
- 3 Slices of Tomato
- 1 Thinly Sliced Onion
- ½ Cup Micro Greens (Or Spinach)
- Salt and Pepper
- ¼ Tsp Garlic Powder

PREPARING THE DISH

1. Put a skillet on medium heat. Once the pan is hot, add a little grass fed butter. Once melted, crack in your eggs and season with salt, pepper, and garlic powder. When the whites start to set, pop the yolk, wait one more minute, then flip. Cook for another two minutes or until they're cooked to your liking.

2. While the eggs are cooking, grab a bowl and throw in the avocado and sriracha. Add a pinch of salt and mix until smooth and creamy. Toast your two pieces of bread and spread your avocado mayo over them. Take one of your eggs and put it on a piece of toast. Next, place your tomatoes, then another egg, the micro greens, the onion slice, and finally the last egg. Top with the second piece of toast, then cut in half and enjoy.

BREAKFAST BANANA PANCAKES, EGGS AND CHIVES

INGREDIENTS

- 2 Cups Organic All-Purpose Flour (Or Flour of Choice)
- ¼ Cup Organic Granulated Sugar
- 4 Tsp Baking Powder
- ¼ Tsp Baking Soda
- ½ Tsp Salt
- 1 ¾ Cups Raw Milk
- ½ Cup Grass Fed Butter
- 2 Tsp Pure Vanilla Extract
- 4 Large Egg
- 2 Bananas
- ½ Tsp Cinnamon
- 4 Tbsp Organic Maple Syrup
- 2 Tsp Chopped Chives
- 1 Tbsp Milk
- Butter
- Salt and Pepper

PREPARING THE DISH

BATTER

1. Mix together the flour, sugar (or sweetener), baking powder, baking soda, and salt in a large-sized bowl. Make a well in the centre and add the milk, melted butter, 1 egg, and vanilla. Use a whisk to mix the wet ingredients together. Then slowly mix them into the dry ingredients. Mix until smooth. If you find the batter is too thick, mix in a little extra milk until reaching desired consistency. Put to the side and let it rest while heating up your skillet.

2. Heat a skillet over low-medium heat, then use a little butter to lightly grease the pan. Pour 1/4 cup of batter onto the pan and spread out gently into a round shape with the back of your measuring cup (or whatever utensil you are using). When it is golden brown and bubbles begin to pop on the surface, flip with a spatula and cook until golden brown.

3. Place a small saucepan on medium heat. Take the 2 bananas and cut them in half long ways, then into 1/2 inch pieces. Put the bananas into the pan with cinnamon and maple syrup. Heat up for about 4 min. When done, top the pancakes with the banana mixture.

EGGS

4. Heat up a skillet on medium heat. Scramble the three remaining eggs in a bowl with a tablespoon of milk and a dash of salt. Put a little butter in the pan and add the eggs once the butter has melted. Use a spatula and push the eggs inwards from the edges until your eggs are the desired consistency. Plate the eggs and top with the chives.

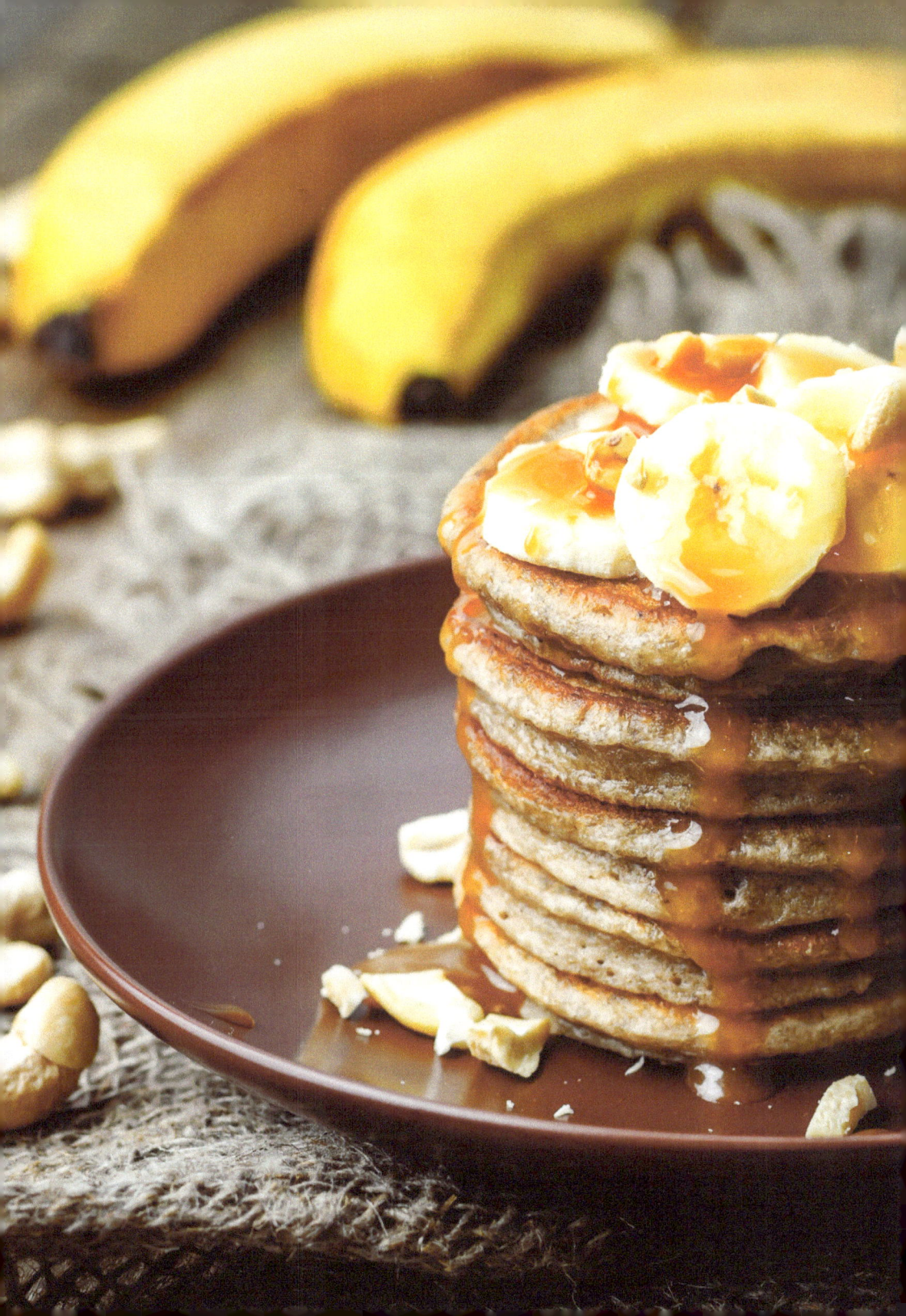

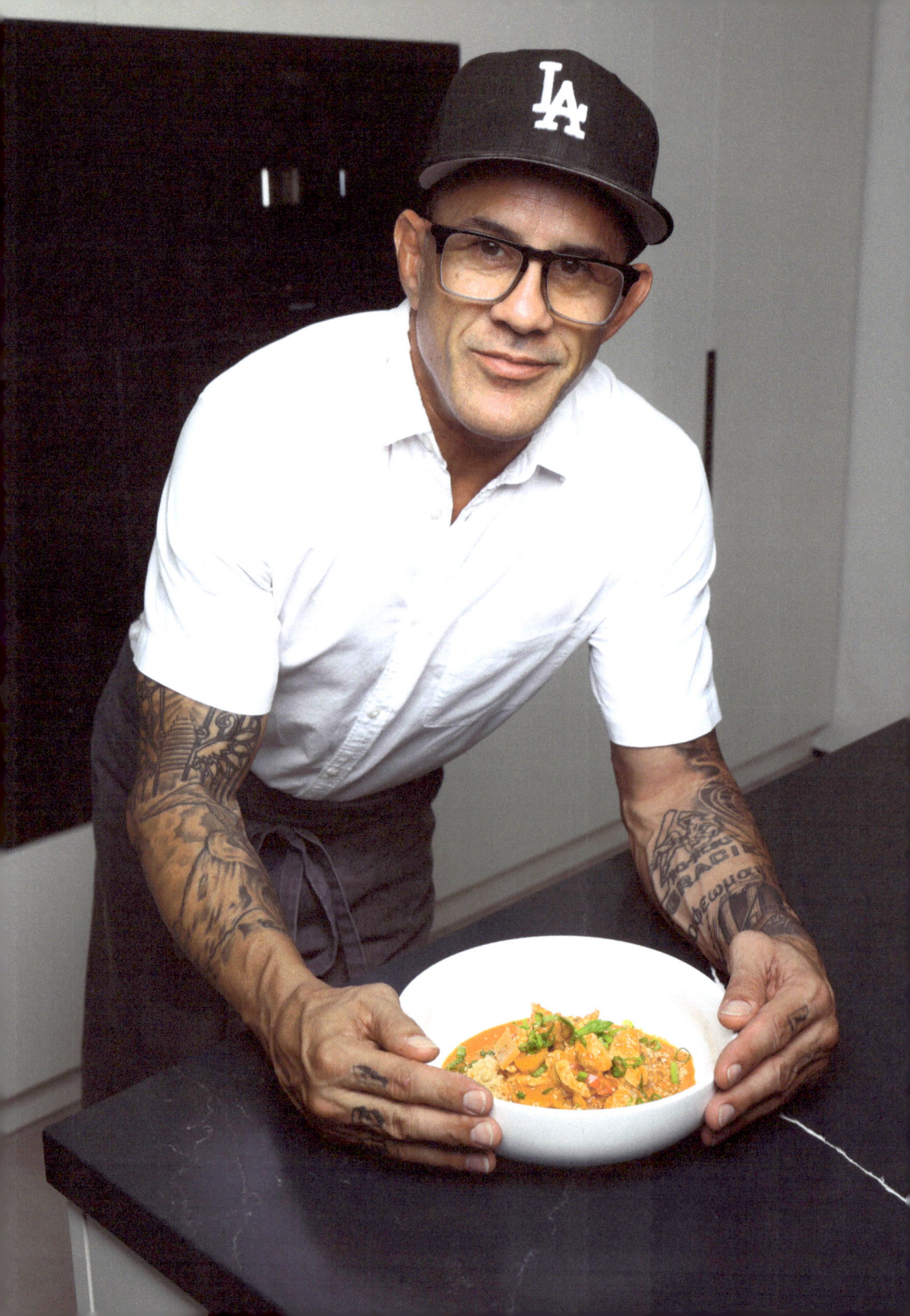

MAIN COURSES

SHRIMP AND GARLIC PASTA

INGREDIENTS

- 3 Tbsp Unsalted Grass Fed Butter
- 2 Tbsp Olive Oil
- 2 lb Large Shrimp, Peeled And Deveined
- 4 Garlic Cloves, Minced
- ½ Tsp Salt
- ¼ Tsp Black Pepper
- 1 Tsp Red Pepper Flakes (Optional)
- ½ Cup White Wine
- 1 ½ Tbsp Lemon Juice
- ½ Cup Fresh Parsley, Chopped
- ½ lb Pasta

PREPARING THE DISH

1. Bring a pot of water to a boil and cook pasta al dente, about 8–10 min.

2. In a skillet, add butter and olive oil over medium-high heat. After the butter has melted, add the raw shrimp and cook until pink and opaque, turning the shrimp occasionally. Now add the garlic cloves, salt, pepper, and red pepper flakes. Stir together until the garlic becomes fragrant, about 1–2 min. Bring the heat to high and pour in the white wine and fresh lemon juice. Let it come to a quick boil, then turn heat off.

3. Plate and garnish the shrimp scampi with freshly chopped parsley. Serve over hot buttered pasta.

AVOCADO CHICKEN SALAD

INGREDIENTS

- 2 Medium Cooked Chicken Breasts, Shredded or Chopped
- 2 Ripe Avocados, Diced
- ¼ Cup Roasted Corn
- ¼ Cup Red or Green Onion, Minced
- 1 Tbsp Cilantro, Finally Chopped
- ½ Tsp Garlic Powder
- 2 Tbsp Lime or Lemon Juice
- 1 Tbsp Olive Oil
- Smoked Paprika
- Salt and Pepper

PREPARING THE DISH

1. Preheat oven to about 400°.
2. Season chicken with salt, pepper, and garlic powder, then place in baking dish. Cook in oven for 15–18 minutes or until done. Using a meat thermometer, check the internal temperature to be around 165°F. When the chicken is done, let it sit for 5 minutes to cool, then either cut it into pieces or shred.
3. In a large bowl, add the shredded/chopped chicken, avocado, onion, corn, and cilantro.
4. Drizzle with the lime juice and olive oil, then season with salt, pepper, garlic powder, and a little smoked paprika. Toss gently until all the ingredients are combined.

CHICKEN PASTA SALAD

INGREDIENTS

- 1 lb Fusilli Pasta
- 2 Boneless Skinless Chicken Breasts (About 1 Pound)
- 1 Tsp Garlic Powder
- Salt and Black Pepper
- 1 Tbsp Extra Virgin Olive Oil
- 4 Slices Bacon (Cooked and Crumbled)
- 2 Cup Halved Grape Tomatoes
- 2 Cup Spinach, Packed
- ½ Cup Crumbled Feta
- ¼ Red Onion (Thinly Sliced)
- 2 Tbsp Freshly Chopped Dill or Basil

DRESSING

- 1/4 Cup Extra-Virgin Olive Oil
- 3 Tbsp Red Wine Vinegar
- 1/2 Tsp Italian Seasoning
- 1 Clove Garlic Minced
- 1 Tbsp Dijon Mustard
- Salt and Black Pepper

PREPARING THE DISH

1. Fill a pot with water, add salt, and bring to a boil. Cook pasta until al dente, about 8–10 min. Drain and transfer to large bowl.

2. Cut chicken breasts into small cubes and season with garlic powder, salt, and pepper. Get a skillet and put it on medium heat. Cook chicken until cooked through, about 8 minutes. Let rest 10 minutes.

3. Meanwhile, make dressing: In a medium bowl, whisk together olive oil, vinegar, Italian seasoning, garlic, and mustard. Season with salt and pepper.

4. In the large bowl with the pasta, throw in all of the other ingredients. Pour dressing over salad, toss until coated, and serve.

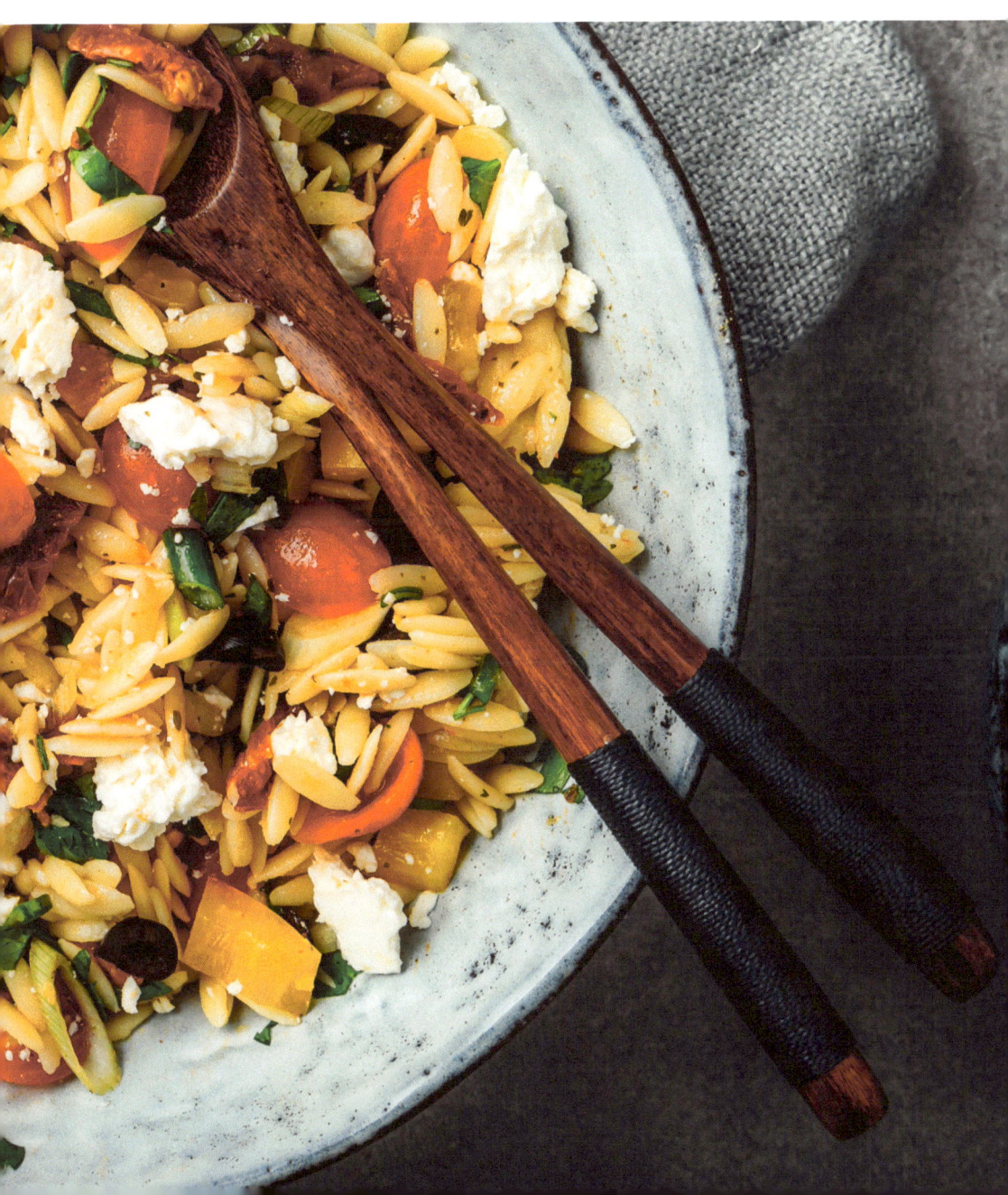

SALMON POKE

INGREDIENTS

- 1 Cup Sushi Rice
- 1 Cup Water
- 3 Tsp Rice Vinegar
- ½ Tsp Salt
- 7 Oz Wild-Caught Salmon Fillet (Sushi Grade)
- 2 Tbsp Low Sodium Soy Sauce
- 2 Tbsp Lemon Juice
- ½ Avocado (Thinly Sliced)
- ½ Cucumber (Halved Lengthwise and Sliced)
- 2 Tbsp Pickled Ginger
- 1 Green Onion (Thinly Sliced)
- 5 Small Sheets of Nori
- 1 ½ Tsp Raw Honey
- ¼ Tsp Toasted Sesame Seeds
- ¼ Tsp Black Sesame Seeds

PREPARING THE DISH

1. Add the rice to a fine mesh strainer and submerge in a bowl filled with water. Shake the rice a few times to remove excess starch. Transfer the rice to a medium pot and add 1 cup of water. Cover the pot and bring to a boil over medium-high heat. Once boiling, reduce the heat to medium-low and simmer for 10 minutes. Remove the pan from the heat and let stand for 15 minutes. Remove the lid and fluff the rice with a fork or rice paddle. Transfer the rice to a large bowl.

2. Mix together the rice vinegar, sugar, and salt and pour over the rice while still hot. Gently fold the rice to incorporate. Cover and set aside until ready to assemble the bowl.

3. Cut the salmon fillet into ½-inch cubes. It may be easier to slice if you place the salmon in the freezer for a few

minutes to help it firm up.

4. Just before assembly, place the salmon in a bowl and season with the soy sauce and lemon juice.

5. To assemble, place a few spoonfuls of rice into a medium bowl. Top the rice with the seasoned salmon, avocado, cucumber, ginger, green onions, nori sheets, toasted sesame seeds, and black sesame seeds.

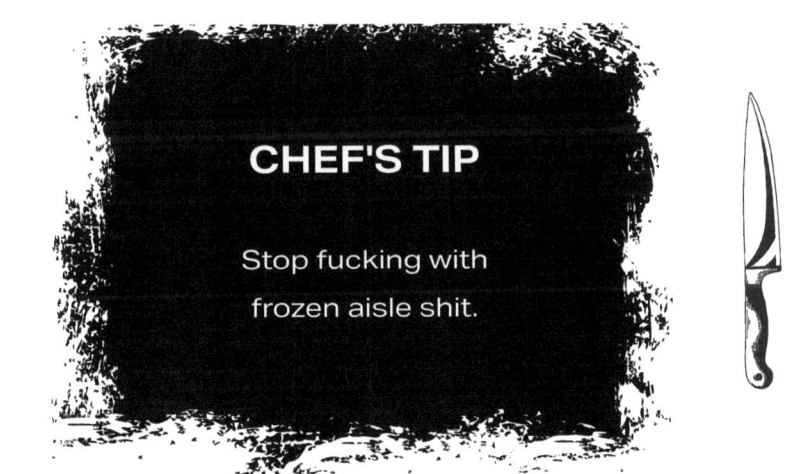

CHEF'S TIP

Stop fucking with frozen aisle shit.

PAN SEARED OVEN FINISHED SALMON WITH ROASTED VEGGIES

INGREDIENTS

- 2 5-Ounce Salmon Fillets
- 2 Tbsp Olive Oil
- 1 Lemon (Juiced)
- 2 Cup Broccoli Florets (Cut In Half)
- 2 Cups Cremini Mushrooms
- 2 Cups Sweet Potato (Chopped)
- 1 Zucchini (Sliced And Quartered)
- 1 Red Bell Pepper (Chopped)
- 1 Red Onion (Chopped)
- 2 Tbsp Olive Oil
- 2 Tbsp Balsamic Vinegar
- 4 Cloves Garlic, Minced
- 1 ½ Tsp Dried Thyme
- Salt and Pepper

RECOMMENDED FRESH HERBS FOR SALMON
- Chives
- Tarragon
- Parsley
- Thyme

PREPARING THE DISH

1. Pre-heat the oven to 400°.
2. Pre-heat a non-stick skillet over medium-high heat and season the salmon with salt and pepper. Add some olive oil to the skillet and place the salmon in the pan skin side down. Sear for 2 minutes on each side, then transfer to the oven for 6–7 minutes, or until firm to the touch. Remove from oven and plate the salmon.

3. Finely chop fresh herbs and sauté with 2 tablespoon grass fed butter in a skillet for three minutes or until herbs become aromatic. Squeeze lemon over herbs and serve over the salmon.

4. Preheat oven to 425°. Lightly oil a baking sheet. Place broccoli florets, mushrooms, sweet potato, zucchini, bell pepper, and onion in a bowl and add olive oil, balsamic vinegar, garlic, and thyme. Add salt and pepper to taste. Gently toss to coat all the veggies. Place into oven and bake for 15 minutes or until tender and caramelized. When done, serve 1 1/2 cups along side one piece of salmon.

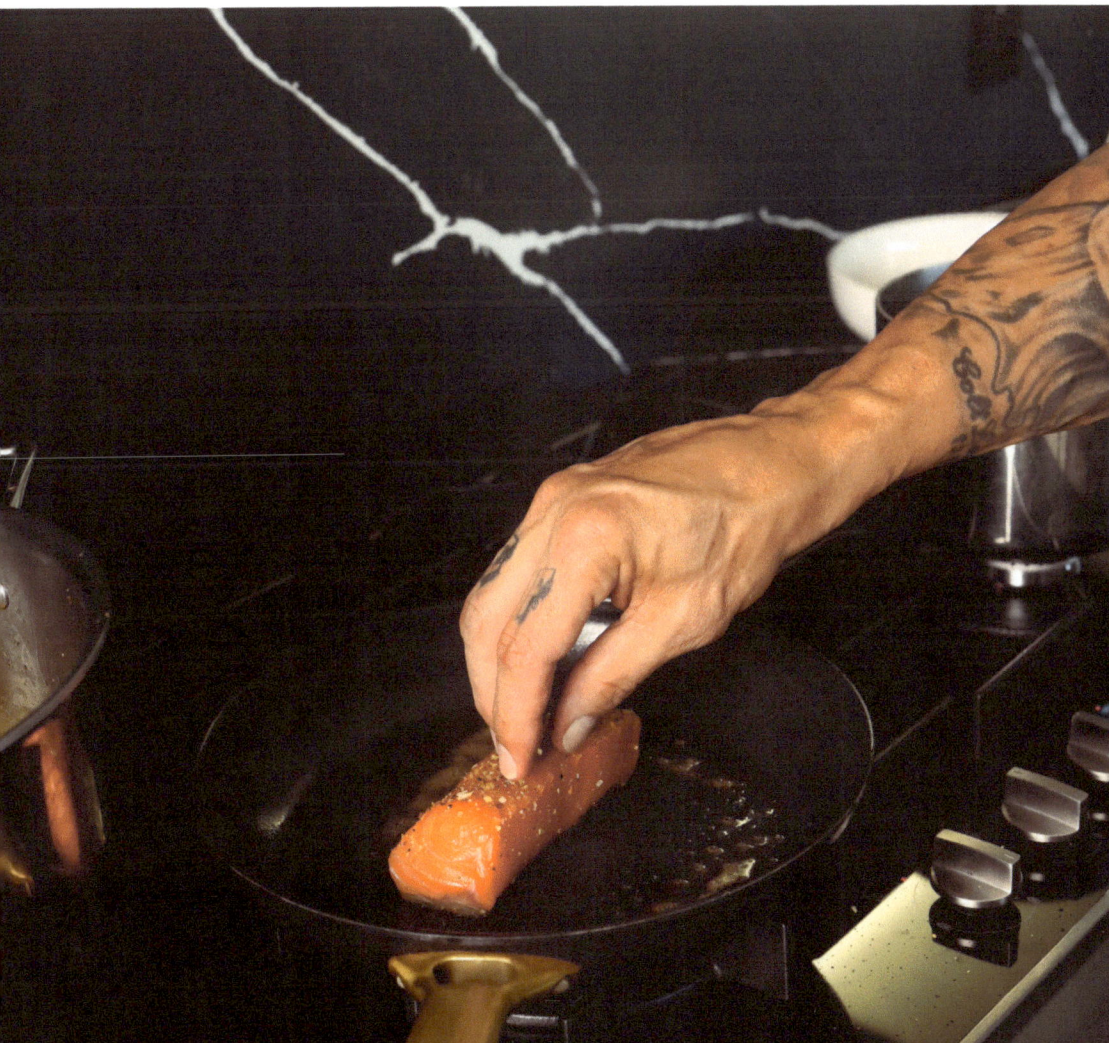

BROCCOLI WITH BEEF

INGREDIENTS

- 1 Pound Flank Steak (Sliced Into 1/4 Inch Thick Strips)
- 3 Cups Small Broccoli Florets
- ½ Cup Beef Broth
- 5 Cloves Garlic (Minced)
- 1 Tbsp Sesame Oil
- ¼ Cup Chopped Green Onion
- 2 Tsp Sesame Seeds
- 1 Tbsp Minced Ginger
- 1 Tsp Corn Starch
- 1 Cup White Rice

SAUCE

- ¼ Cup Raw Honey (Or Preferred Sweeter)
- ½ Cup Low Sodium Soy Sauce
- 1 Tsp Corn Starch

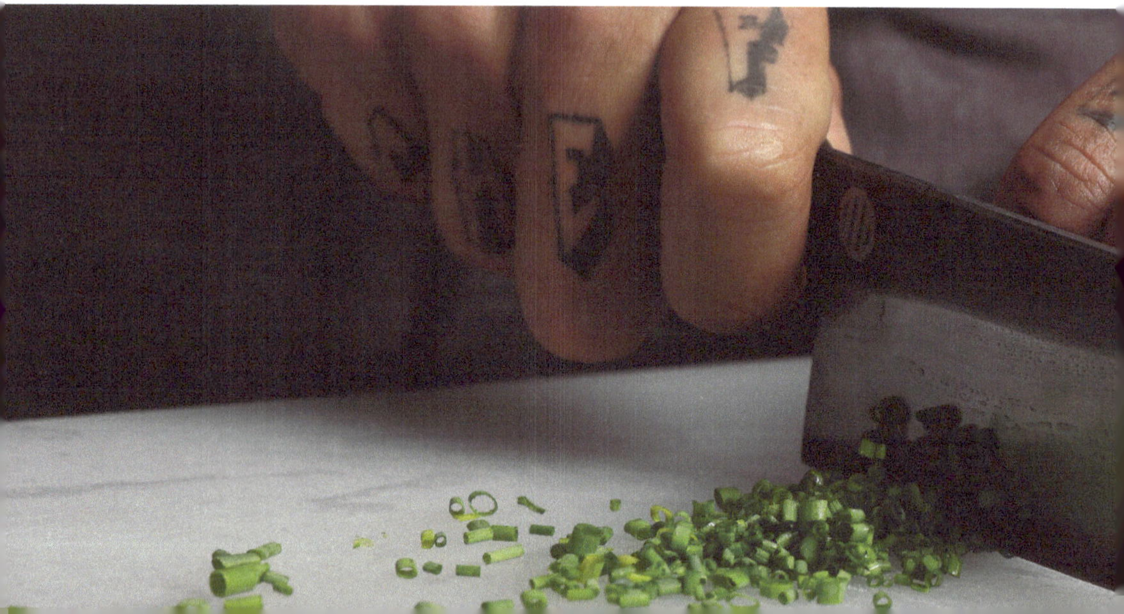

PREPARING THE DISH

1. In a large bowl, toss the sliced beef with the sesame oil until well-coated. When done, set aside.

2. Heat a skillet over medium heat until hot. Add sliced beef and cook until it browns, stirring frequently. Transfer beef to plate.

3. While beef is cooking, steam broccoli until tender. Add broccoli florets, garlic, ginger, and corn starch to a skillet and stir. Add beef broth. Stirring occasionally, simmer until broccoli is tender, about 10 minutes. Meanwhile, proceed to the next step to prepare sauce.

4. Stir together all sauce ingredients in a bowl until well-mixed.

5. When broccoli is tender, return beef to pan and pour sauce on top. Add green onion and sesame seeds. Stir until everything is coated with sauce. Simmer for about 5 minutes to thicken the sauce. Serve over 1 cup of white rice.

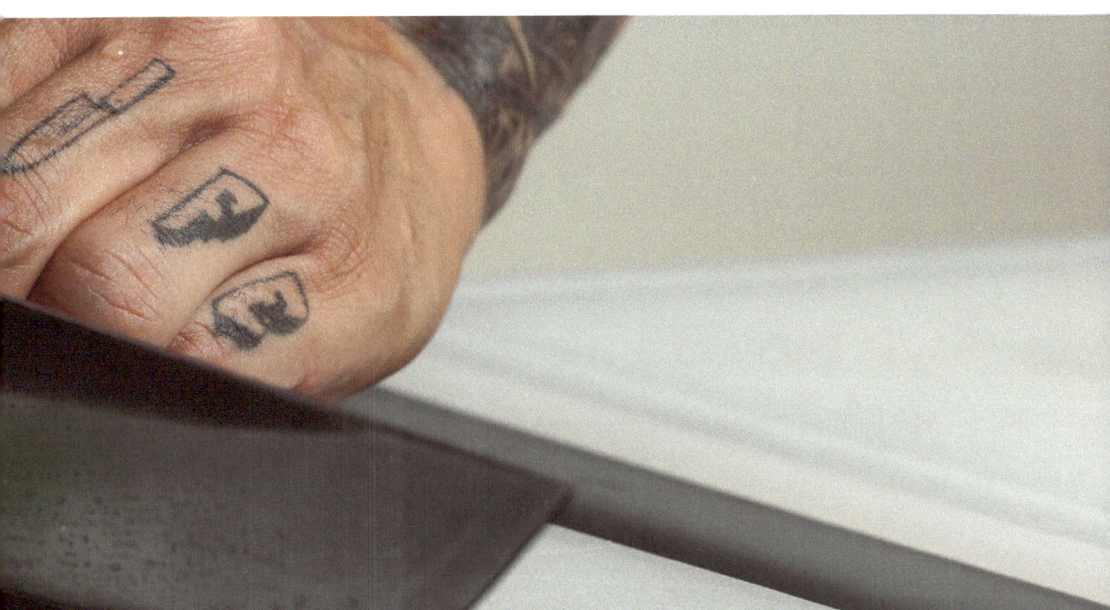

ORANGE CHICKEN OVER QUINOA

INGREDIENTS

- 1 lb Boneless, Skinless Chicken Breasts, Cut Into Bite-Sized Pieces
- Salt and Pepper
- 2 Tbsp Sesame Oil
- Orange Chicken Sauce (Ingredients Below)
- Thinly-Sliced Green Onions
- Toasted Sesame Seeds
- Orange Zest
- Any Vegetable You Would Like To Add

SAUCE
- 3 Cloves Garlic, Minced
- ½ Cup Fresh Orange Juice
- ½ Cup Honey
- ⅓ Cup Soy Sauce
- ¼ Cup Rice Wine Vinegar
- 3 Tbsp Cornstarch (Optional)
- ½ Tsp Ground Ginger
- ½ Tsp White Pepper
- Zest Of One Orange
- Pinch Of Crushed Red Pepper Flakes

QUINOA (OPTIONAL - YOU CAN USE RICE AS WELL)
- 1 Cup Dry Quinoa
- 2 Cups Chicken Broth

PREPARING THE DISH

1. Season chicken generously with salt and pepper.

2. Heat oil in a large saute pan over medium heat. Add chicken and saute for about 4–6 minutes, stirring occasionally, until the chicken is nearly cooked through.

3. While the chicken is cooking, whisk all the ingredients for the sauce together until combined. If you would like the sauce to be even sweeter, add an extra 2–4 tablespoons of raw honey.

4. Add the orange chicken sauce into the pan with the chicken, and stir to combine. Let the sauce come to a boil, then boil for an additional minute or two until thickened. Remove from heat and serve immediately over quinoa or rice. Top with green onions, sesame seeds, and additional orange zest.

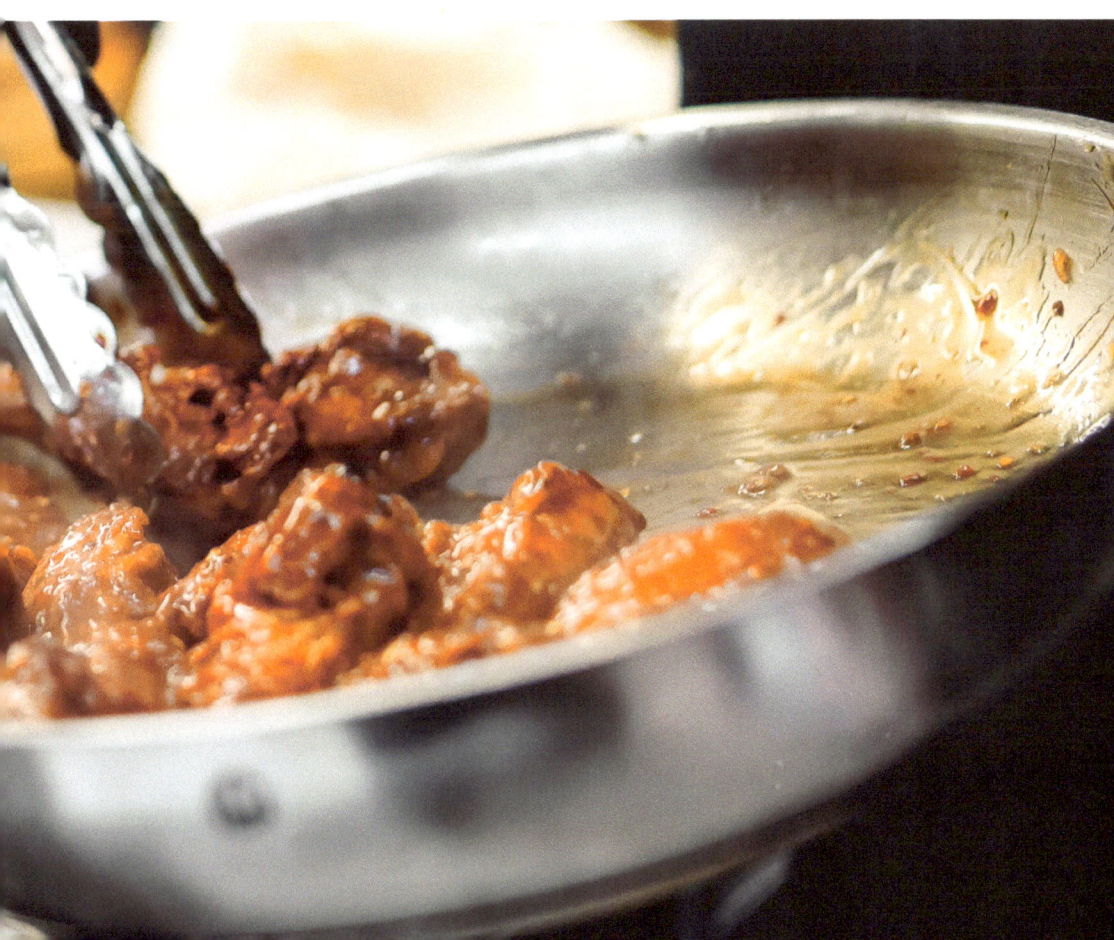

HEALTHY TURKEY CHILI

INGREDIENTS

- 1 lb Lean Ground Turkey
- 1 Onion, Diced
- 1 Bell Pepper (Any Color), Diced
- 1 Can Crushed Tomatoes, Undrained, (Stewed Tomatoes Work Too)
- 1 Can Organic Black Beans
- I Can Organic Kidney Beans Or Garbanzo Beans (Undrained)
- 2 Cups Chicken Broth
- 2 Tbsp Tomato Paste
- 1 Can Chopped Green Chilies
- 1 ½ Tbsp Chili Powder (Or To Taste)
- 1 Tbsp Ground Cumin (Or To Taste)
- Season With Preferred Amount Of Garlic Salt and Pepper

PREPARING THE DISH

1. Heat a large skillet over medium-high heat and cook ground meat until no longer pink.
2. While that is cooking, add onion and bell pepper to a large pot and sauté until soft. Then add the cooked turkey and combine all other ingredients with onion and bell pepper, bring to a boil, decrease heat, and simmer for about 30 minutes or until it thickens. Once it thickens, it's ready to serve.

SALMON CAKES

INGREDIENTS

- 3 Teaspoons Extra-Virgin Olive Oil (Halved)
- 1 Small Onion (Finely Chopped)
- 1 Stalk Celery (Finely Diced)
- 2 Tbsp Fresh Parsley (Chopped)
- 1 ½ Cups Fresh Cooked Salmon (Boneless)
- 1 Large Egg (Scrambled)
- 1 ½ Tsp Dijon Mustard
- 1 ¾ Cups Gluten Free Bread Crumbs
- ½ Tsp Freshly Ground Pepper
- 1 Lemon (Cut Into Wedges)

PREPARING THE DISH

1. Preheat oven to 450°.
2. Coat a baking sheet with grass fed butter or olive oil.
3. Heat 1 1/2 teaspoons oil in a large skillet over medium-high heat. Add onion and celery. Cook and stir until softened (about 3 min). Mix in parsley and turn off heat.
4. Place cooked salmon in a medium bowl. Remove skin, if any, and flake apart with a fork. Add egg and mustard then continue to mix together. Add the onion mixture, breadcrumbs, and pepper. Incorporate thoroughly. Shape the mixture into 8 patties, about 2 1/2 inches wide.
5. Heat remaining oil in the skillet over medium heat. Add 4 patties at a time and cook until the undersides are golden (2–3 min), using a spatula turn them over onto the baking sheet.
6. Bake the salmon cakes until golden on top and heated through (about 15 min). Serve salmon cakes with sauce of choice, and a side of grilled or steamed veggies and lemon wedges.

QUINOA AND SQUASH SALAD WITH CRANBERRIES, PECANS, AND PEARS

INGREDIENTS

- Protein Of Your Choice Is Optional
- 5 Oz Cooked Chicken Breast (Cut Into Bite-Sized Pieces)
- 1 Cup Quinoa
- 1 ¾ Cups Chicken Broth
- 1 Delicata Squash, Cut In Half Lengthwise, De-Seeded, and Cut Into ½" Slices
- ¼ Tsp Cinnamon
- ¼ Tsp Salt
- ¼ Tsp Pepper
- 1 Tbsp Olive Oil
- ½ Cup Pecans (Chopped)
- ⅓ Cup Dried Cranberries (Chopped)
- 1 Pear (Diced)
- 2 Tbsp Chopped Herbs Of Your Choice (I've Used Parsley, Oregano, Sage and Thyme)

DRESSING

- ½ A Lemon (Juiced)
- 3 Tbsp Apple Cider Vinegar
- ½ Tsp Dijon Mustard
- 1 Tsp Pure Maple Syrup
- ½ Tsp Dried Thyme
- ¼ Tsp Salt
- ¼ Tsp Pepper
- 2 Tbsp Olive Oil

PREPARING THE DISH

1. Preheat oven to 400°.

2. In a medium saucepan, bring chicken broth to a boil. Add quinoa, a pinch of salt, and stir. Cover and reduce heat to low. Cook for about 15 minutes, until all liquid is absorbed. Set aside to cool.

3. Line a baking sheet with parchment paper. Place squash on baking sheet and toss with olive oil, cinnamon, salt, and pepper. Roast for 20 minutes or until tender and golden.

4. In a small bowl, whisk together the lemon, apple cider vinegar, dijon, maple syrup, dried thyme, salt, pepper, and olive oil. Season to taste with more salt and pepper. Set aside.

5. To assemble the salad, toss cooled quinoa, pecans, dried cranberries, chopped pear, and a few tablespoons of the dressing. Add the squash and gently toss again. Add herbs and toss once more. Drizzle on more dressing and serve with more to taste.

STEAK AND EGGS WITH CHILI VERDE

INGREDIENTS

- 1 lb Skirt Steak
- Himalayan Pink Salt
- Freshly Ground Black Pepper
- Small Bunch Of Parsley
- 1 Garlic Clove (Finely Minced)
- 1 Lemon
- 1 Tbsp Capers (Finley Minced)
- ½ Tsp Crushed Red Pepper Flakes
- ½ Tsp Raw Honey
- ½ Cup Extra-Virgin Olive Oil (Plus More For Pan)
- 4 Large Eggs

PREPARING THE DISH

1. Cut skirt steak into pieces about 6" long. Pat steak dry with paper towels, then season generously all over with pink Himalayan salt (or salt of choice) and freshly ground pepper. Let rest at room temperature while you make the salsa verde.

2. Pick leaves and tender stems from 1 bunch of parsley and finely chop to make 3/4 cup. You can mix it up with any flavorful leafy greens you have on hand—cilantro, dill, watercress, and/or arugula. Add the greens to a medium bowl. Finely mince 1 garlic clove and 1 tsp lemon zest into the bowl. Squeeze 1 lemon half into bowl (about 4 tsp). Coarsely chop 1 Tbsp capers and add it in. Mix in 1/2 tsp red pepper flakes, 1/2 tsp raw honey, and 1/2 cup extra-virgin olive oil. Season with salt. Set aside until ready to serve.

3. Heat a large cast-iron skillet on high. Dab steaks dry again with paper towels. You want them to be as dry as possible; this will help you get the nice brown crust you're after. Rub extra-virgin olive oil all over the steak, just enough to lightly coat.

4. Once the skillet is hot, gently lay steak in it. Cook 2–3 minutes. Turn steak and cook until second side forms a golden brown crust (about 2 minutes longer). General rule is that once it has a nice sear, it's already perfectly cooked. When done, let steak rest 10 min.

5. While steak rests, pour enough oil into skillet to coat the bottom of the pan, then heat over medium. Immediately crack 4 large eggs into pan — you don't need to wait for the oil to heat up because there's already a lot of residual heat in the pan from when you cooked the steak. Cook eggs until edges are crispy, whites are set, and yolks are still runny, 4–6 minutes. season with salt.

6. Slice steak against the grain, then transfer to a platter. Set eggs alongside steak. Drizzle salsa verde over steak and eggs. Serve remaining salsa verde alongside.

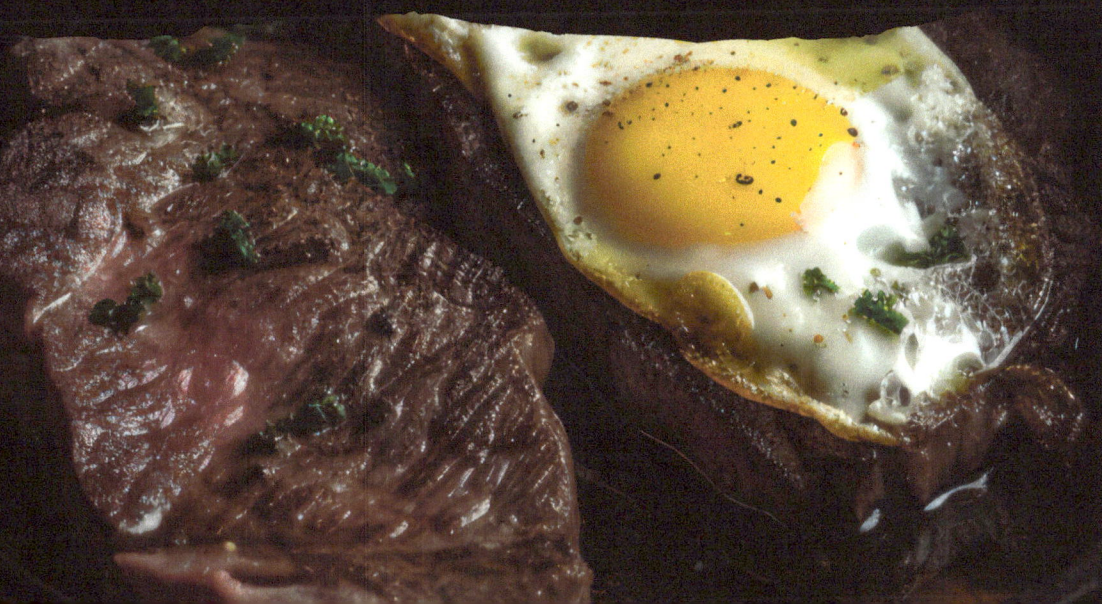

LASAGNA

INGREDIENTS

- 1 lb Organic Sweet Italian Chicken Sausage
- ¾ lb Lean Ground Beef
- ½ Cup Minced Onion
- 2 Cloves Garlic (Crushed)
- 1 (28 Ounce) Can Crushed Tomatoes
- 2 (6.5 Ounce) Cans Canned Tomato Sauce
- 2 (6 Ounce) Cans Tomato Paste
- ½ Cup Water
- 2 Tbsp Raw Honey
- 4 Tbsp Fresh Parsley (Chopped And Divided)
- 1 ½ Tsp Dried Basil Leaves
- 2 Tbsp Fresh Basil (Finely Chopped)
- 1 ½ Tsp Salt (Divided, Or To Taste)
- 1 Tsp Italian Seasoning
- ½ Tsp Fennel Seeds
- ¼ Tsp Ground Black Pepper
- 12 Lasagna Noodles
- 16 Oz Ricotta Cheese
- 1 Egg
- ¾ lb Mozzarella Cheese, Sliced
- ¾ Cup Grated Parmesan Cheese

PREPARING THE DISH

1. Cook sausage, ground beef, onion, and garlic in a large pot oven over medium heat until well browned.

2. Stir in crushed tomatoes, tomato sauce, tomato paste, and water. Season with raw honey, 2 tablespoons parsley, dry basil, fresh basil, 1 teaspoon salt, Italian seasoning, fennel seeds, and pepper. Cover and let simmer for about 1 1/2 hours, stirring occasionally.

3. Bring a large pot of lightly salted water to a boil. Cook lasagna noodles in boiling water for 8–10 minutes. Drain noodles, and rinse with cold water.

4. In a mixing bowl, combine ricotta cheese with egg, remaining 2 tablespoons parsley, and 1/2 teaspoon salt.

5. Preheat the oven to 375°.

6. To assemble, spread 1 1/2 cups of meat sauce in the bottom of a 9x13-inch baking dish. Arrange 6 noodles lengthwise over meat sauce. Spread with 1/2 of the ricotta cheese mixture. Top with 1/3 of the mozzarella cheese slices. Spoon 1 1/2 cups meat sauce over mozzarella, and sprinkle with 1/4 cup Parmesan cheese.

7. Repeat layers, and top with remaining mozzarella and Parmesan cheese. Cover and bake in the preheated oven for 25 minutes. Remove the foil and bake for an additional 25 minutes.

8. Rest lasagna for 15 minutes before serving.

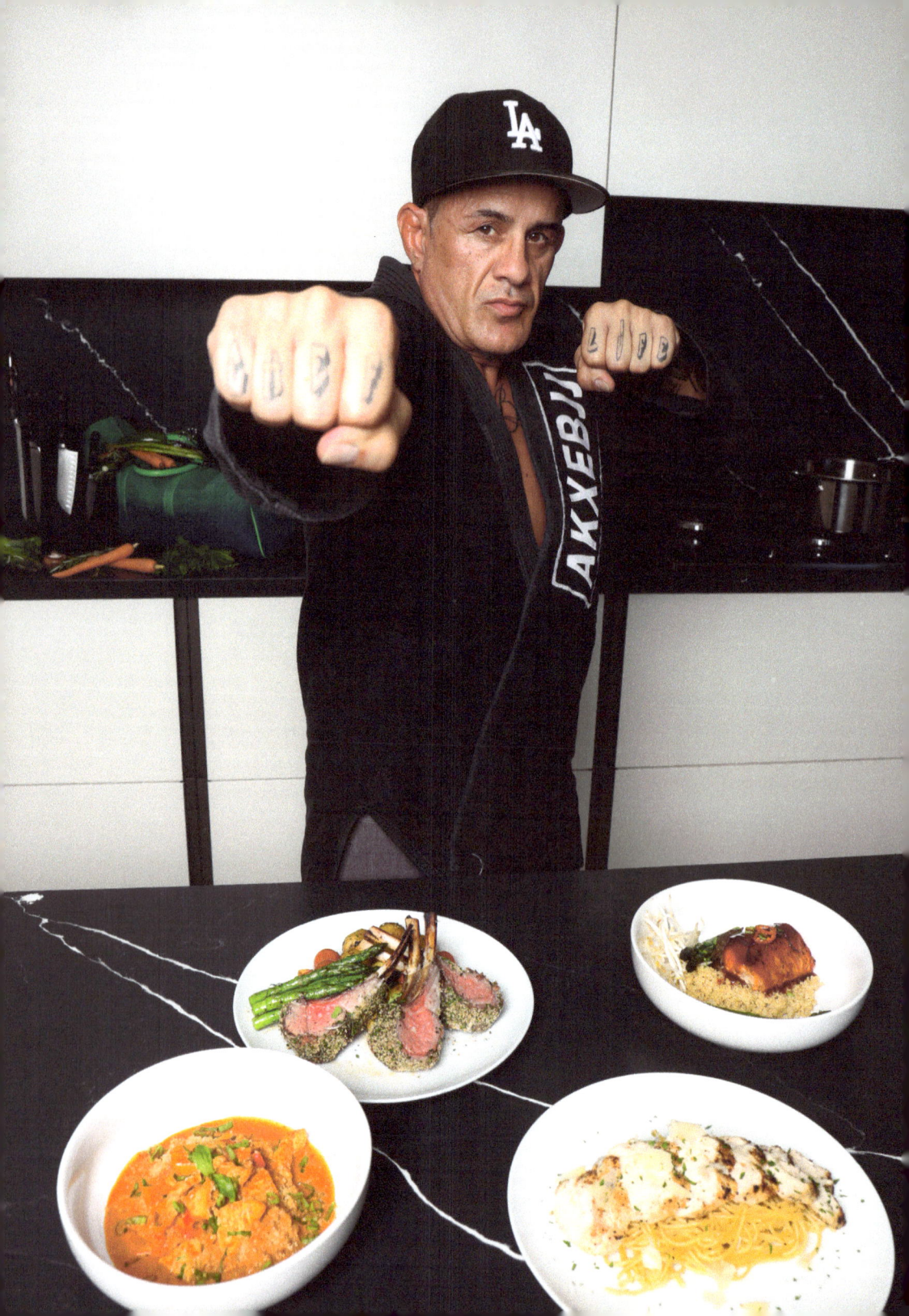

SIGNATURE DISHES

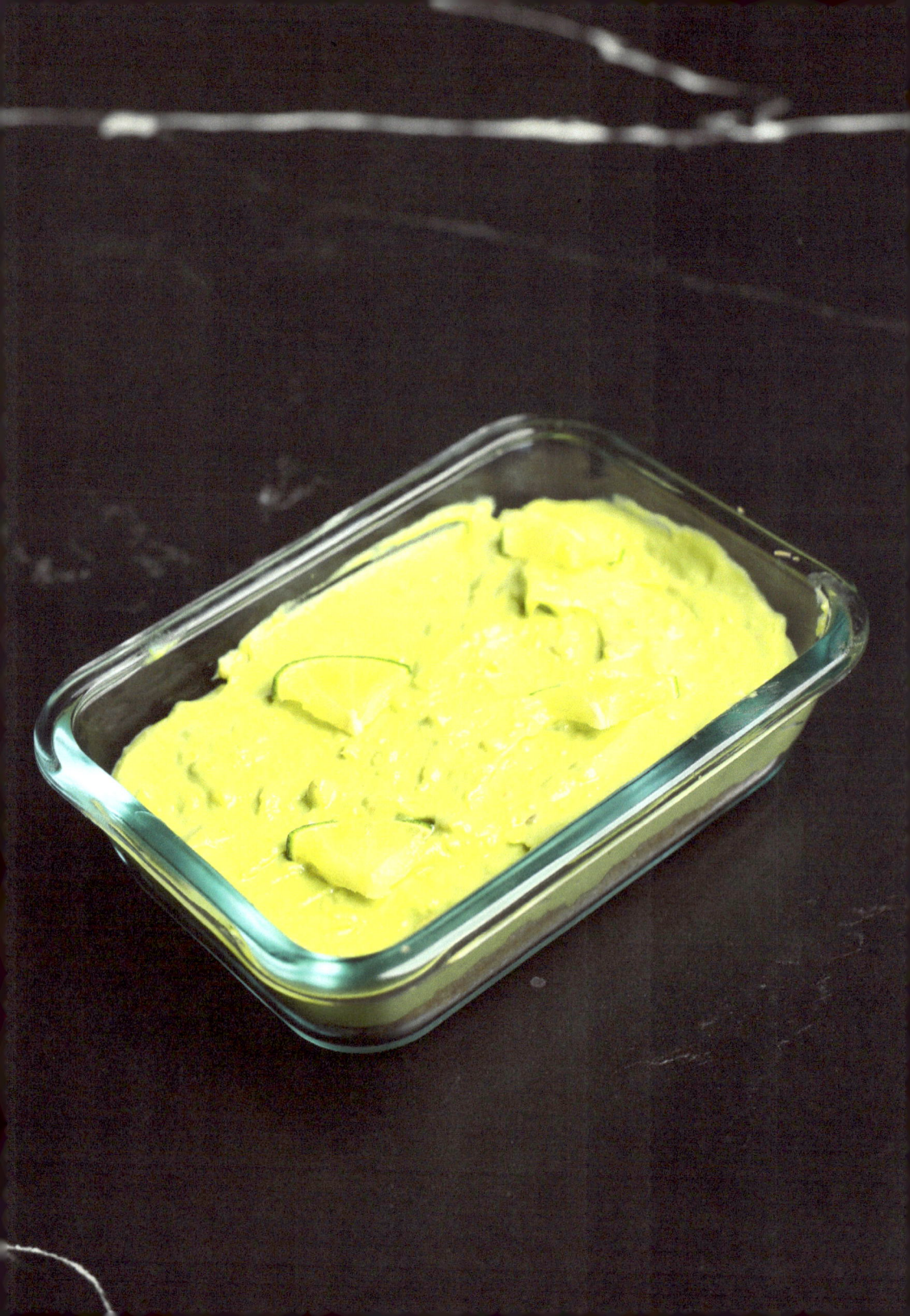

LOVATO N' LIME — DEMI LOVATO'S AVOCADO LIME CHEESECAKE

INGREDIENTS

CRUST
- 3 Oz Pecans
- ½ Cup Shredded Coconut
- 3 Tbsp Cacao Nibs
- 2 ½ Tbsp Cocoa Powder
- 3 Oz Pitted Dates
- 1 Tbsp Coconut Oil

FILLING
- 1 lb Avocado Flesh (4–5 Medium Avocados)
- ½ Cup Coconut Cream
- 5 Limes, Zested And Juiced (You Need ½ Cup Lime Juice)
- ½ Cup Pure Organic Maple Syrup
- ¼ Cup Cold Pressed Coconut Oil
- 2 Limes (Zest For Topping)

PREPARING THE DISH

1. Start with the crust.
2. Preheat the oven to 350°.
3. Line an 8-inch (20cm) springform cake pan with parchment paper.
4. Place the pecans and shredded coconut on a parchment paper lined baking sheet. Place in the oven for 3–5 minutes, until toasted. Be careful not to burn the shredded coconut.
5. Transfer the pecans and coconut to a food processor. Add the cacao nibs, cocoa powder, dates, and coconut oil and process until the mixture is crumbly. It should hold together when pinched. If not, add more dates, one by one, and process again.
6. Transfer the mixture to the prepared cake pan and press into the bottom. Refrigerate while making the filling.
7. Place the lime zest, lime juice, avocados, coconut cream, maple syrup, and coconut oil into the food processor. Process until smooth. Taste and add more lime juice or maple syrup, if desired.
8. Pour the filling over the crust. Chill in the refrigerator for a minimum of 4 hours..
9. Zest two limes over the cake and serve. I recommend that this be eaten within a couple days.

I once prepared the avocado cheesecake for a family gathering at Demi's place. Her mother and sisters were present, and I served the dessert with a sprinkle of the crust on top and adorned it with flowers. The response was overwhelmingly positive, and Demi and her family loved the creation. From then on, the avocado cheesecake became a favorite for Demi, and she would often request it.

LOVATO N' LIME

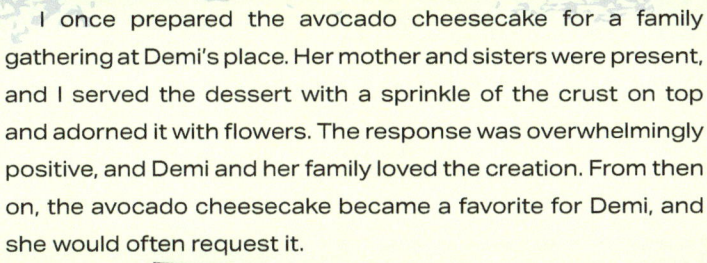

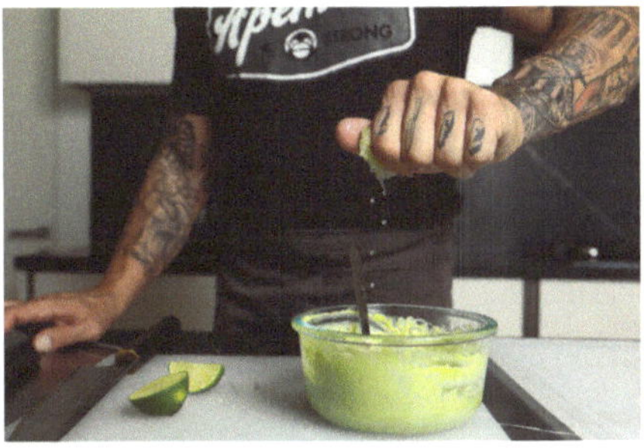

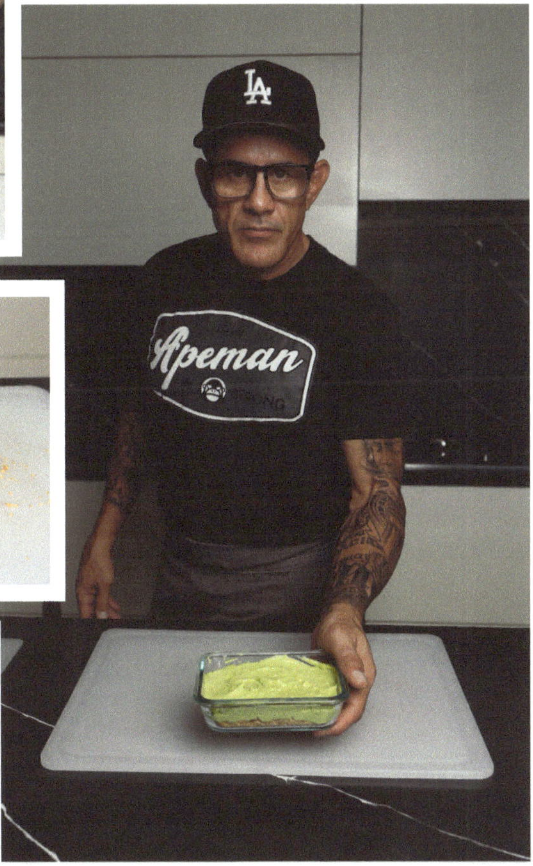

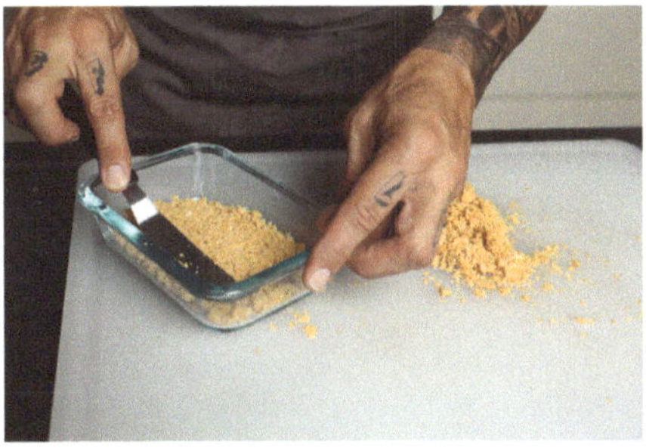

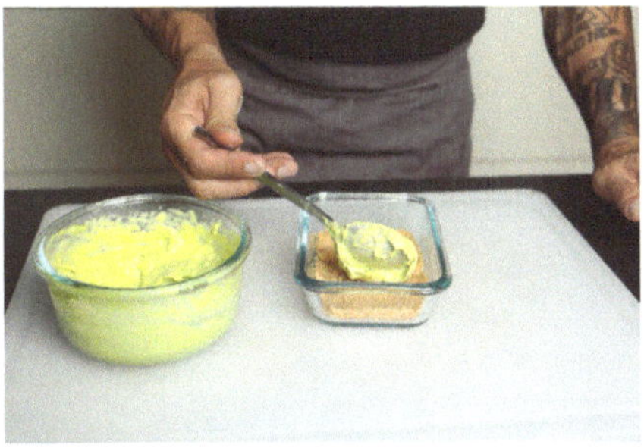

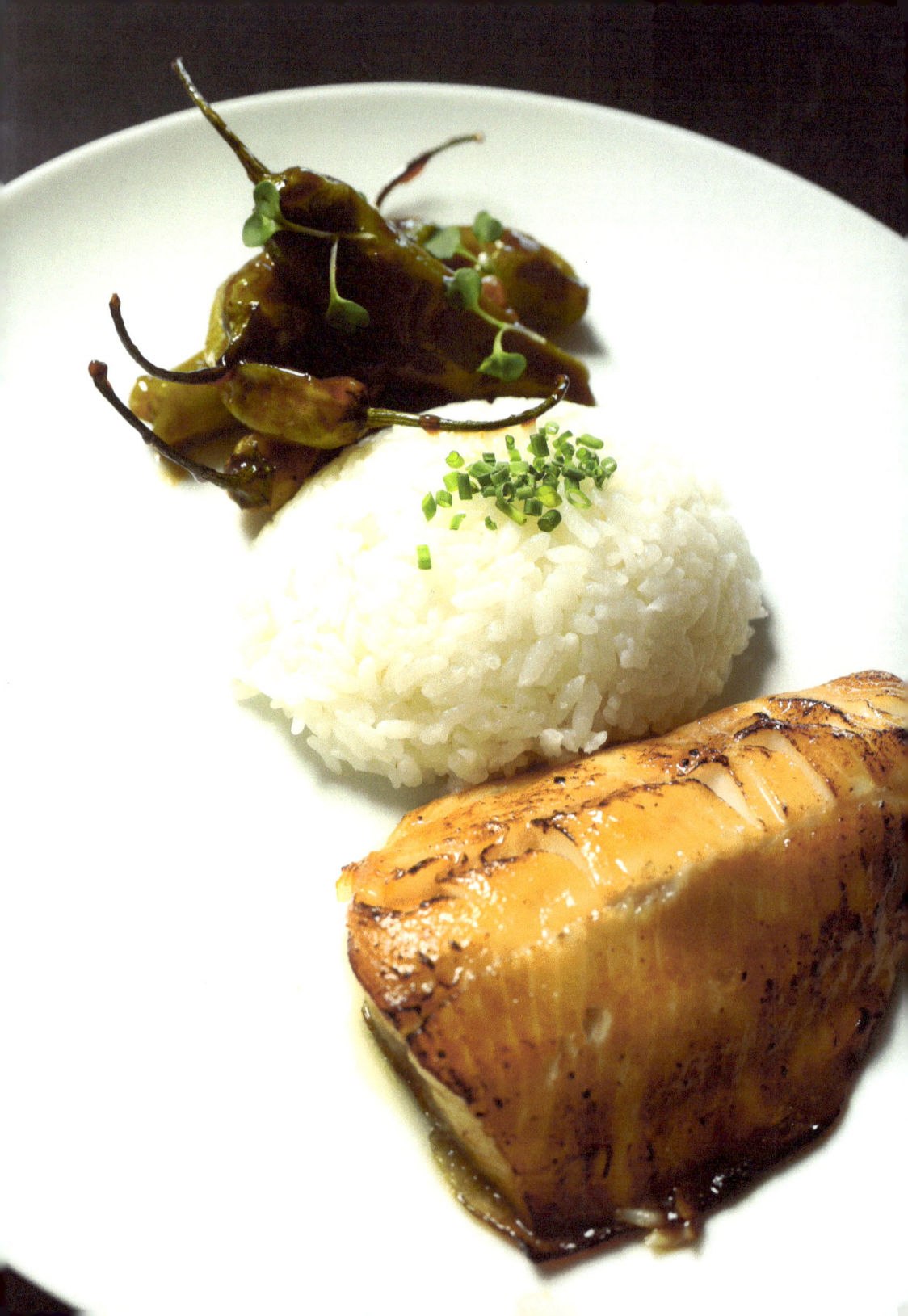

KSI BLACK COD OVER JASMINE RICE

INGREDIENTS

- ¼ Cup Sake
- ¼ Cup Mirin
- ¼ Cup Black Fermented Miso Paste (Or Regular Miso)
- 3 Tbsp Raw Honey
- 4 (8-oz) Black Cod Fillets
- 1 Cup Cooked Jasmine Rice
- Green Onion (Chopped)

PREPARING THE DISH

1. Bring the sake and mirin to a boil in a medium saucepan over high heat. Boil for 20 seconds to evaporate the alcohol. Turn the heat down to low, add the miso paste, and whisk. When the miso has dissolved completely, turn the heat up to high again and add the raw honey. Keep whisking for another minute. Take off heat and let cool to room temperature.
2. Dry the cod with a paper towel thoroughly. Cover the fish with the miso marinade and place in a non-reactive dish or bowl and cover super tight with plastic wrap. Let it marinade for at least 24 hours, but up to 3 days.
3. When ready to cook, preheat oven to 400°.
4. Heat an oven-proof skillet over high heat on the stovetop. Lightly wipe off any excess miso clinging to the fillets, but don't rinse it off. Put a little oil in the pan, then place the fish skin-side-up on the pan and cook until the bottom of the fish browns and blackens in spots, about 3 minutes. Flip and continue cooking until the other side is browned, 2 to 3 minutes. Transfer to the oven and bake for 5–10 minutes, until fish is opaque and flakes easily.
5. Add the cooked fillets onto cooked Jasmine rice and garnish with green onion.

KSI BLACK COD

KSI's reaction to the black cod was priceless. The moment he entered the room, the aroma greeted him, and he immediately recognized the dish he adored. His heartfelt appreciation and excitement filled the air, and I knew I had hit the mark in satisfying his taste buds while keeping his nutritional needs in mind.

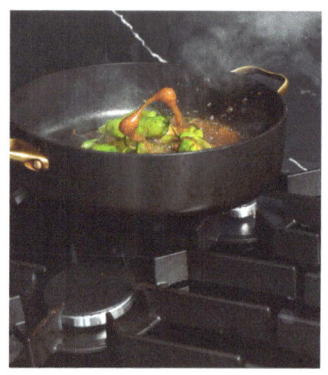 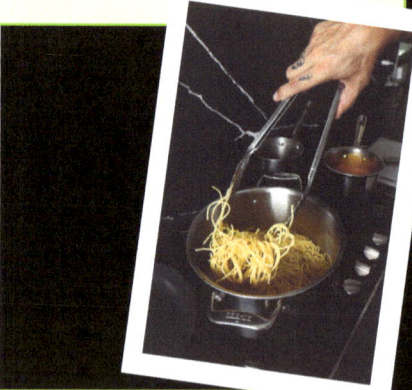

His love for simple comfort food, particularly butter noodles, held a special place in his heart as it reminded him of his mom's cooking from his childhood. I made sure to recreate this dish in a healthier way, using raw Parmesan cheese and grass-fed butter, aligning it with his training diet.

LOGAN'S NOODLES

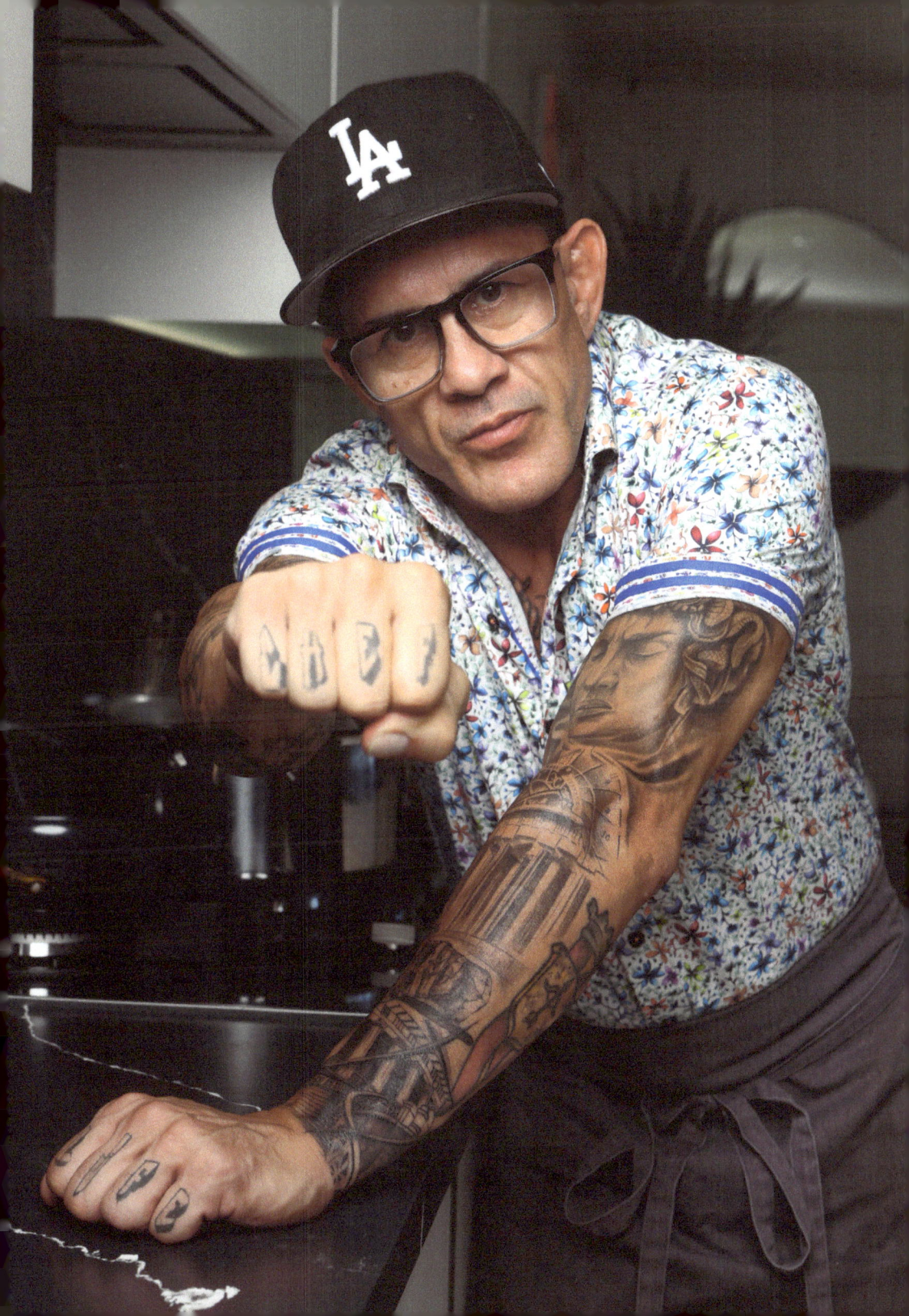

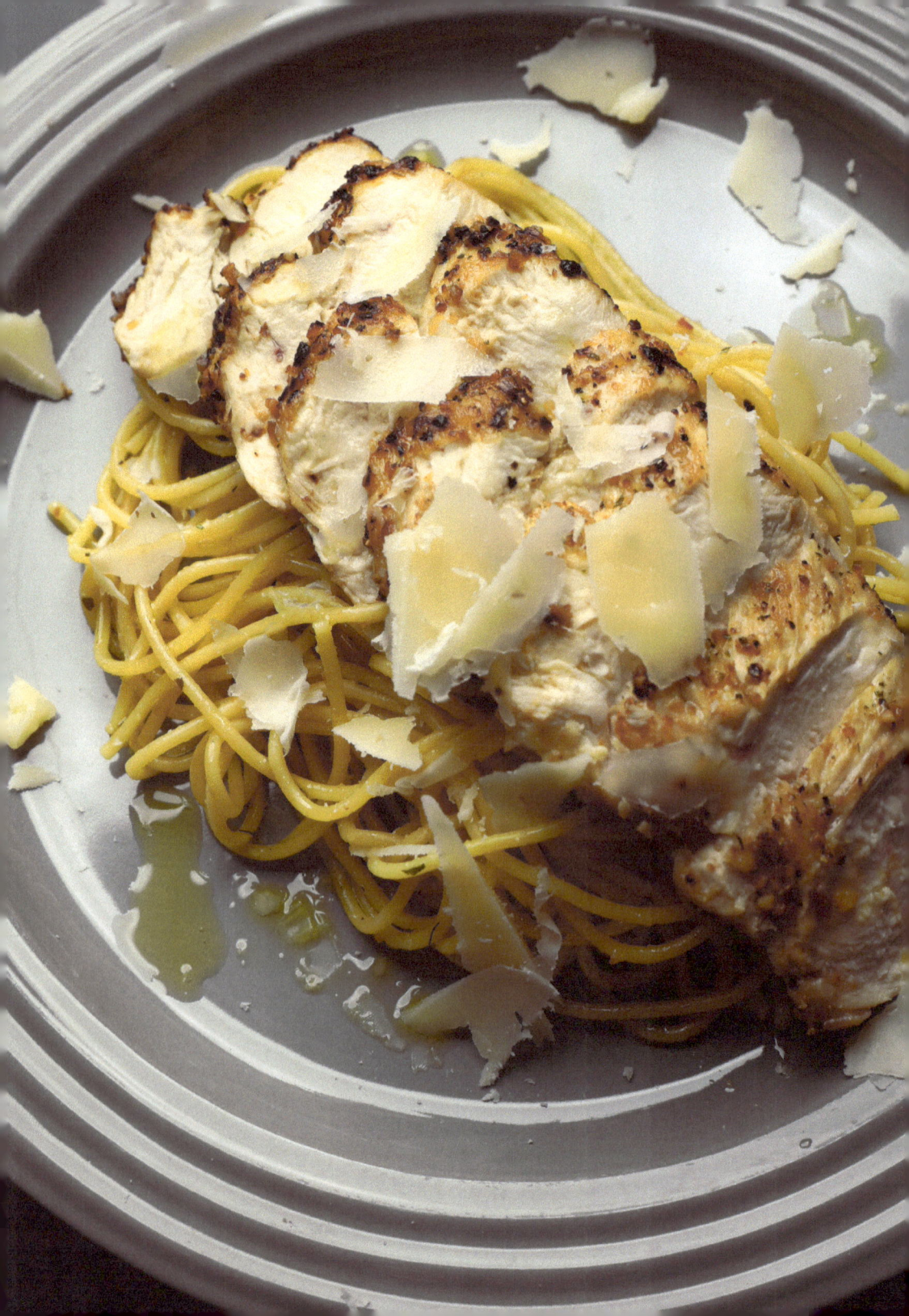

LOGAN PAUL'S BUTTER NOODLES WITH BAKED HERB CHICKEN BREAST

INGREDIENTS

- 1 Package (16 Oz) Spaghetti Noodles
- 6 Tbsp Grass Fed Butter
- ⅓ Cup Raw Grated Parmesan Cheese
- Salt and Ground Black Pepper
- 6 Oz Organic Chicken Breast
- 2 Tsp Herbs De Province
- 3 Cloves Of Garlic

PREPARING THE DISH

1. Fill a large pot with lightly salted water and bring to a boil. Put the pasta in water and bring back to a boil. Cook the pasta al dente, around 8 minutes. Drain and return pasta to pot. Melt butter into the noodles and add 3 cloves chopped garlic to it. Sauté on the low heat for about five minutes. Mix butter, garlic, parmesan cheese, salt, and pepper into pasta until evenly combined.
2. Preheat oven to 450°.
3. Coat the chicken with a little bit of olive oil and then season the chicken with the herbs de province and a little bit of salt. Place the chicken breast in a baking dish, and cook in the oven for 15–18 min, or until the chicken is cooked through. The time will depend on how thick the chicken breast is. I would recommend using a meat thermometer: the thickest part of the breast should measure 165°F.
4. Once cooked, remove the chicken from the oven, slice into thin pieces, and serve over the top of the pasta.

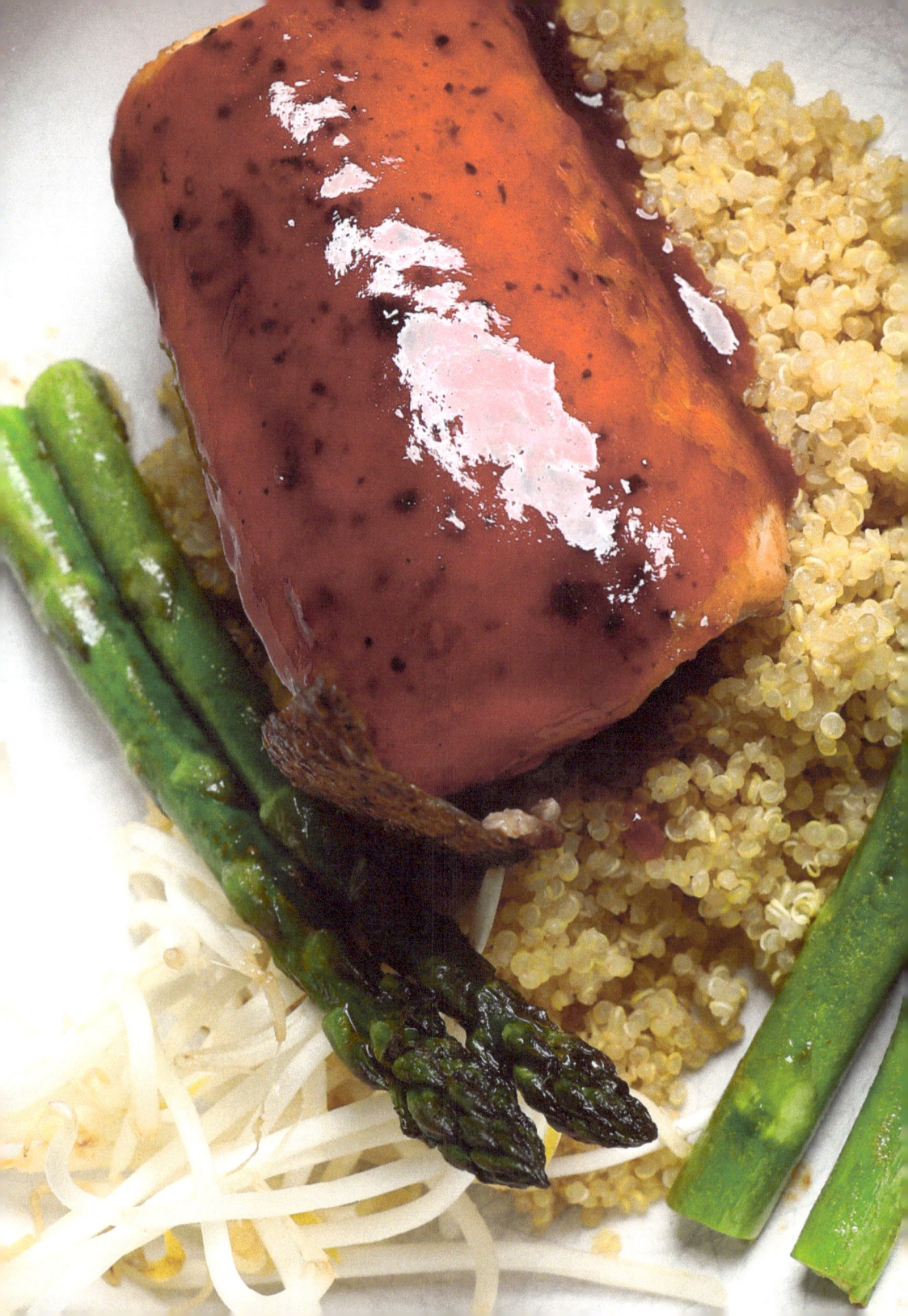

DK SALMON — HONEY AND FERMENTED GOCHUJANG GLAZED SALMON

INGREDIENTS

- 2 (6-Oz) Boneless Salmon Fillets
- 3 Tbsp Fermented Gochujang
- 1 Tbsp Raw Honey
- 1 Tsp Fresh Lime Juice
- Toasted Sesame Seeds
- Toasted Sesame Oil
- 2 Tbsp Scallions (Finely Sliced)
- 8 Spears Of Asparagus (Steamed)

    GLAZE
- Gochcujang Paste
- Honey
- Dash of Tamari

PREPARING THE DISH

1. In a bowl, whisk together gochujang paste, honey, and a dash of tamari
2. Preheat oven to 400°.
3. Coat your salmon with a little sesame oil and salt, then place on baking sheet. Bake for about 7 minutes, then use a brush and glaze the salmon with the honey gochujang glaze. Bake for another 8 min, then pull it out, glaze it one more time, and let sit for a few minutes.
4. Steam the asparagus for about 5 minutes, then throw in a quick ice bath (blanching). When the asparagus is done, take it out of the ice bath and let it dry off. Cut it in diagonal pieces and put it in a bowl. Pour in a little bit of rice, wine vinegar, some honey, and sesame seeds, mix together, and serve alongside fish and rice.

DK SALMON

One of the coolest things I do is make dishes that each of my individual clients really love. The gochujang glazed salmon is a dish I created for DK. We talked about foods he likes and what flavors he enjoys. He had tried some Korean and Vietnamese food, but not much. DK also likes salmon because it's healthy for his brain.

So, I decided to make something new for him. I used gochujang, which is a chili paste, and mixed it with raw honey to keep things both a little sweet and healthy. The first time he smelled the dish, he was amazed. And when he tasted it, he couldn't believe how good it was. He didn't expect to like these kinds of flavors so much, but the mix of flavors—spicy from gochujang, sweet from honey, and the specific salmon taste—all came together beautifully.

DK was surprised that he could eat something so tasty during his training. He used to think training food had to be boring.

This dish became a favorite for DK. He liked it so much that he asked for it almost every other day. He'd just say "gochujang" and we'd both laugh. It's cool to make food that makes people happy, and it's a reminder of how important it is to understand what someone likes to make them a dish they'll really enjoy.

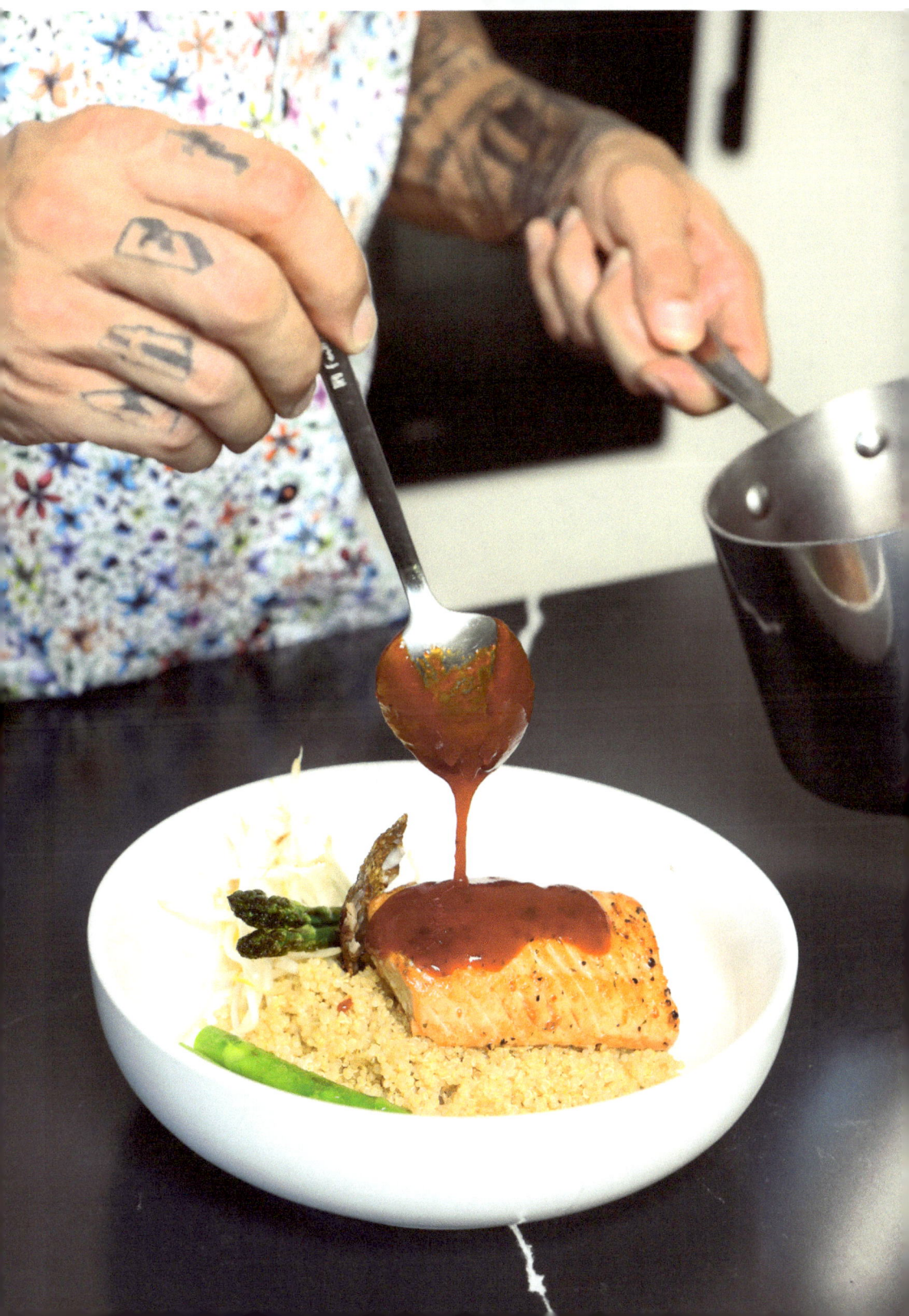

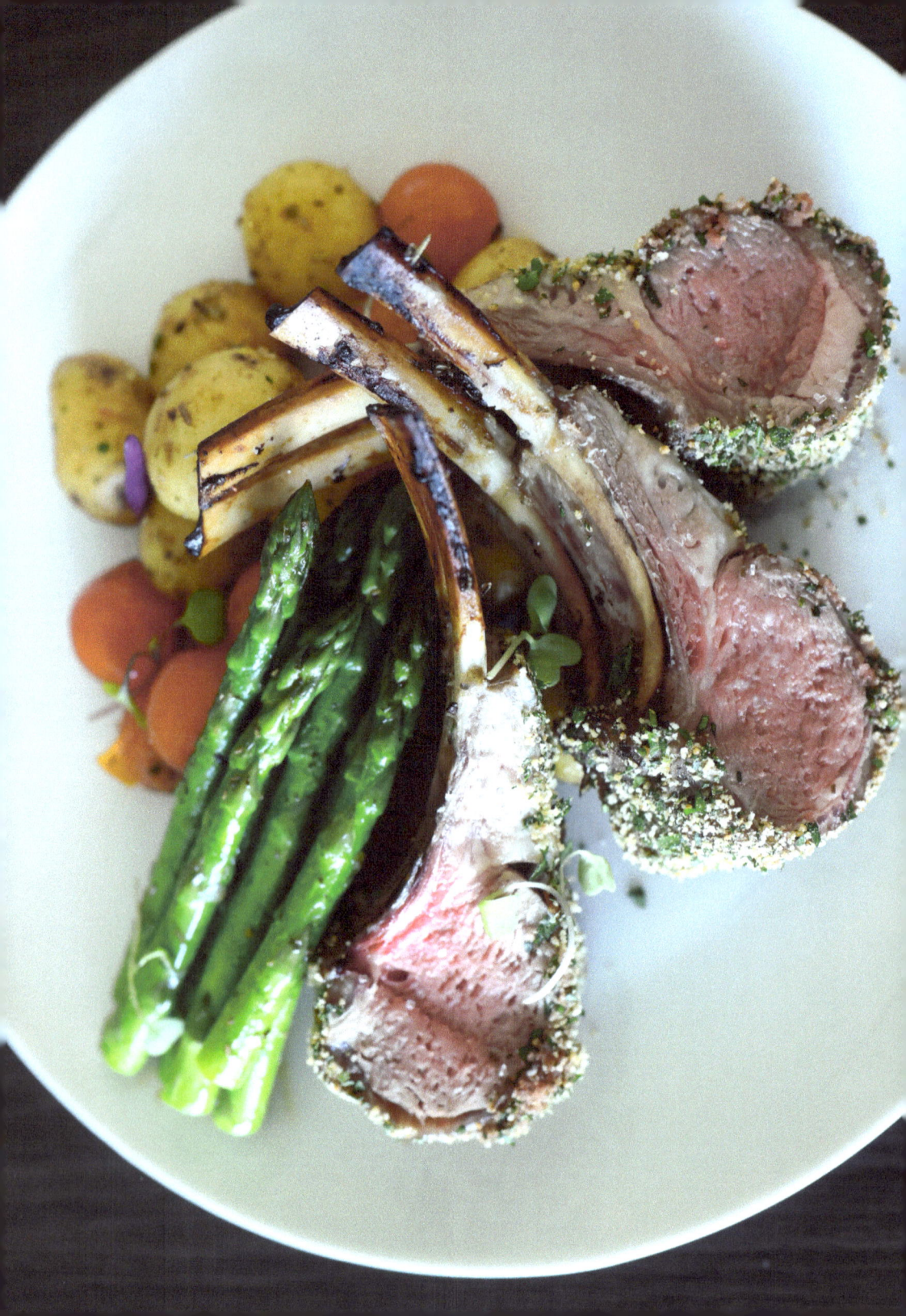

CONOR'S CHOPS — LAMB CHOPS WITH ROASTED BABY POTATOES AND TOMATOES

INGREDIENTS

- 1 Rack Of Lamb (Frenched)
- 1 Bunch Fresh Italian Parsley
- 1 Cup Toasted Bread Crumbs
- 4 Cups Baby Potatoes
- 2 Cups Cherry Tomatoes
- Olive Oil
- Salt And Pepper
- 3 Cloves Garlic (Chopped)
- 1 Tsp Rosemary (Finely Chopped)

PREPARING THE DISH

1. Set lamb out for about an hour to reach room temperature.
2. Preheat oven to 450°.
3. Take baby potatoes and cut them in half. Put them in a bowl, drizzle some olive oil over them, and coat them thoroughly. Do the same with the tomatoes in another small bowl. Once that is done, season with finely chopped rosemary, salt, and pepper. Put a piece of parchment paper on a baking sheet and then put the potatoes and tomatoes on it. Make sure not to over crowd them. Do your best to make sure there is space in between the individual pieces to allow for better roasting. 10 minutes after you start the lamb, put them on the middle rack of the oven (cook for 25 min or until tender).
4. Once the lamb has reached room temperature, season the lamb rack with lemon juice, salt/pepper and on both sides rub the garlic all over.

5. Roast the lamb close to the top of the oven until the rack of lamb reaches 125°–130° internal temp on a meat thermometer (about 25 min, or longer if you like yours cooked medium or medium-well). Use the thermometer on the thicker part of the rack, and try not to hit the bone. The temperature will go up around 5 more degrees as the lamb is resting.
6. Transfer the rack of lamb to cooling dish, cover with foil, and let rest for about 10 min.
7. While the lamb is cooking, get a blender or food processor and mix together half of the bunch of parsley and breadcrumbs. (If you don't have a blender or food processor, use a knife and finely mince everything together. It might take longer, but you can still get the job done.) Mix until a fine powder is made. You want the mixture green in color, so if it's too light, add more parsley slowly to get a green color. You also do not want it to be moist at all. If you find it's a little moist, then let it sit out until it dries, then re-blend it.
8. After lamb has rested, cut in between the bones and transfer to a plate. Grab the parsley-breadcrumb mixture, take one of the lamb chops, and dip the outer edge into the powder. Roll it so the powder coats the whole outer edge of the lamb chop. Do that with each one, and then plates over roasted baby potatoes and tomatoes.

Cooking for someone as renowned as Conor McGregor was a fantastic experience. I created the Conor McGregor lamb chop dish when he was preparing for the fight against Khabib in Las Vegas. I was staying with Conor and took the chance to chat with him about his food preferences. I wanted to know what kind of dishes he enjoyed, especially during training camp.

Conor shared some thoughts, mentioning foods that reminded him of home and dishes he liked. One day, while shopping, I spotted an impressive rack of lamb chops and remembered that Conor liked lamb. I thought, why not make him something special? I brought the lamb chops home, gave them a nice cut (a process known as Frenching), and started working on a dish that would satisfy his cravings.

For the lamb chops' coating, I took breadcrumbs and parsley, blending them to create a fine powder. It was a simple but delightful reverse crust. After seasoning and roasting the lamb chops, I let them rest before slicing. I coated them in the reverse crust, adding a twist to the classic dish. To complement the lamb, I served rosemary-roasted baby potatoes and cherry tomatoes.

Conor came home from a grueling training session, hungry and ready for a good meal. I plated the lamb chops for him, and as he dug into the dish, a smile spread across his face. About three bites in, he looked at me and exclaimed, "Eric, man, these are amazing." His joy was evident, and it felt fantastic to know that he enjoyed the meal I prepared. The reverse crust was a hit, and the whole combination hit the spot for him.

During training camp, fighters are often focused and don't have much time to indulge. This dish, though simple, brought Conor a moment of pleasure amidst his intense training routine. He even asked for more, but I had to remind him about staying on track. Throughout the camp, I made that dish for him a few more times, and it became a requested favorite.

Knowing that someone of Conor's caliber appreciated my cooking was incredibly satisfying. This experience reminded me of the impact food can have, even in the midst of a fighter's demanding schedule. It was a reminder that a simple, well-prepared meal can bring anyone joy and comfort.

CONOR'S CHOPS

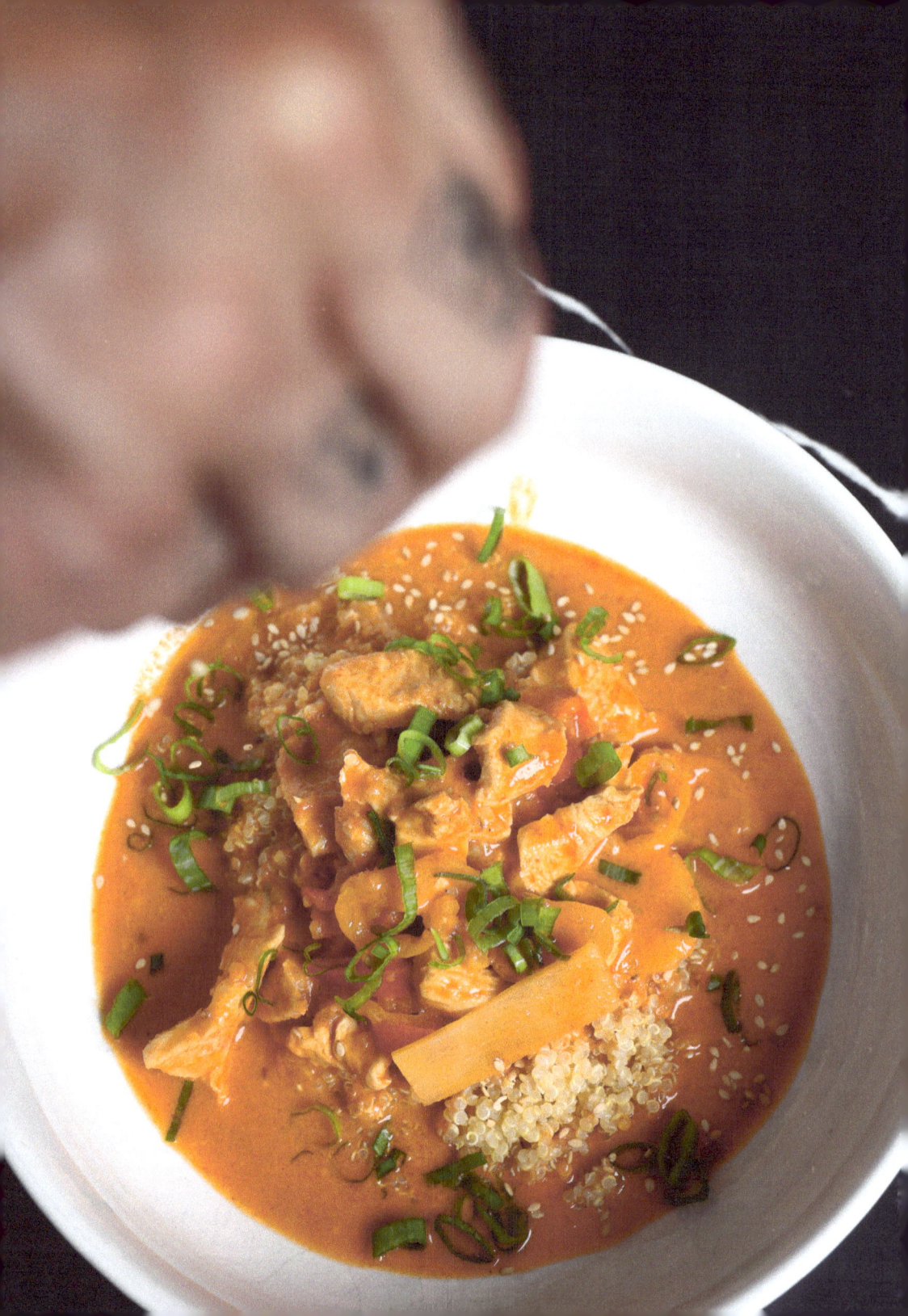

PATRICK'S CURRY — THAI RED CURRY

INGREDIENTS

- 12 Oz Chicken Breast, Cut Into Bite-Size Strips (2 Inch Long, ¼ Inch Wide)
- 2 Tbsp Toasted Sesame Oil
- 4 Tbsp Red Curry Paste (More Or Less, Depending On Your Spice Tolerance)
- ½ Onion Sliced
- ½ Tbsp Garlic, Minced
- 1 Tsp Ginger, Minced
- ½ Tbsp Coriander Stem, Minced (Optional)
- 1 Stalk Lemon Grass (Or Lemon Grass Paste, 1 Tbsp)
- 2 Tsp Fish Sauce
- 1 Tbsp Raw Honey
- 1 Red Bell Pepper, Cut Into Wedges
- 1 Cup Zucchini, Cut
- 1 Can Coconut Milk (Full Fat)
- ½ Cup Stock / Water
- 2 Tsp Lime Juice
- 8-10 Leaves Thai Basil, Chopped Roughly Or Torn

PREPARING THE DISH

1. Heat oil in a skillet. Add sliced onion, minced ginger, and garlic. Saute for a minute, until it is aromatic.
2. Add red curry paste and minced coriander root. Saute for 2–3 minutes, until oil starts oozing out on the side, and you can smell the aroma.
3. Add coconut milk, stock, lemon zest, raw honey, fish sauce, and lemongrass stalk (or paste). Mix well and bring to a boil. Turn the heat down and let simmer for 2–3 minutes.
4. Add chicken and let it simmer for 7–8 minutes. Add the veggies when the chicken is almost cooked. Reduce the sauce almost by half. Cook for another 2 minutes, until the veggies are just cooked but still have a bite.
5. Remove the lemongrass stalk. Add chopped or torn Thai basil.
6. Serve over rice with more garnishing of basil and fresh coriander leaves.

PATRICK'S CURRY

Cooking isn't just about food; it's about stirring up memories and emotions. The story behind Patrick's Thai red curry dish is a perfect example of this delicious connection.

Patrick Minor had traveled to Thailand and loved its local food and street eats. Bangkok and Phuket left a mark on him, and he often reminisced about the vibrant flavors. One day, he returned from the gym feeling sluggish and low on energy. I saw this as a chance to lift his spirits and infuse some vitality into him with a new meal.

Inspired by his Thai memories, I crafted a red curry dish with coconut milk, aiming to capture the essence of his travel experiences. I wanted every bite to whisk him back to those bustling Thai streets and vibrant markets.

Patrick's reaction was the best reward. As he dug into the dish, a grin appeared on his face. He even laughed a little. When I asked what was amusing him, he shared that the curry had taken him right back to Thailand. The flavors were a perfect match, making him feel like he was reliving those Thai adventures.

This dish wasn't just about feeding Patrick; it was about offering a taste of cherished memories. It was humbling to see how a simple plate of food could rekindle past moments and evoke such strong feelings.

Cooking his Thai red curry was a reminder that food is more than just sustenance; it's a bridge to cultures, experiences, and cherished memories. The joy of providing him with a dish that brought back his travels was both heartwarming and motivating. It reinforced my commitment to creating dishes that not only fill the stomach but also resonate with the heart and soul.

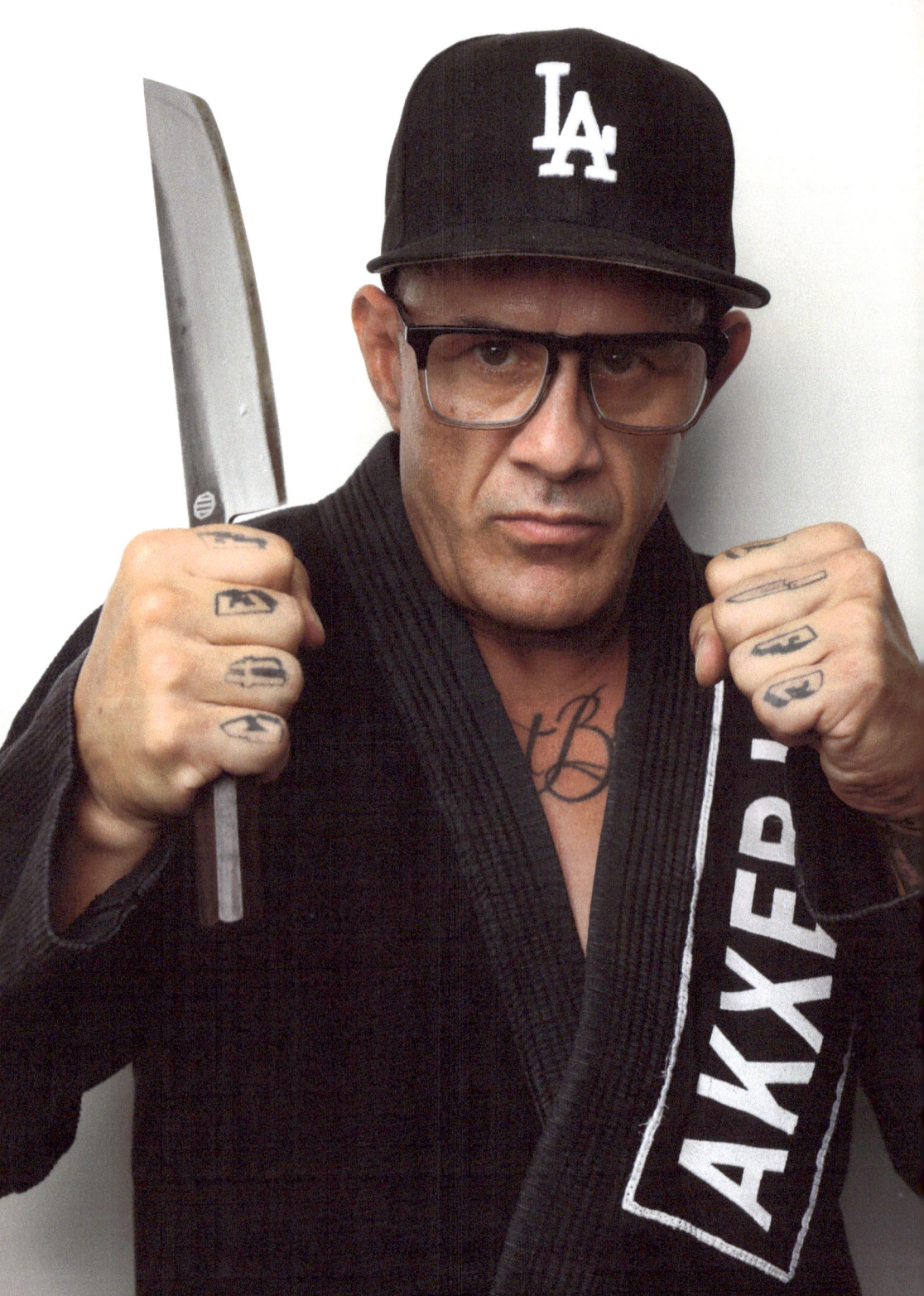

SNACKS

OVERNIGHT CHIA CUPS

INGREDIENTS

- ¼ Cup Cacao Powder Or Unsweetened Cocoa Powder
- 3–5 Tbsp Maple Syrup
- ½ Tsp Ground Cinnamon (Optional)
- 1 Pinch Himalayan Pink Salt
- ½ Tsp Vanilla Extract
- 1 ½ Cups Raw Milk (Or Almond Milk, Light Coconut Milk For Creamier Texture, Or Unsweetened Almond Milk)
- ½ Cup Chia Seeds
- ½ Cup Raspberries

PREPARING THE DISH

1. In a bowl, sift cocoa powder to prevent lumps. Then add maple syrup, ground cinnamon, salt, and vanilla and whisk together. Then whisk in a little milk at a time until a paste forms. Add remaining milk and whisk until smooth. Add the raspberries and chia seeds. Whisk for 2 more minutes. Cover and refrigerate overnight (minimum 5 hours), or until it reaches desired consistency.

2. This will last roughly 4–5 days. Serve cold with whatever toppings you enjoy.

CAPRESE SLIDERS WITH BALSAMIC

INGREDIENTS

SKEWERS
- 1 Pint Cherry Tomatoes
- 1 Medium Ripe Peach (Optional), Pitted and Sliced Into Small, Bite-Sized Pieces No Larger Than Your Tomatoes
- 8 Ounces Ciliegine (Mini Mozzarella Balls)
- 1 Small Bunch Of Basil (Smaller Basil Leaves Are Preferable, You'll Need Between 22–44 Leaves Total)
- 22 Small (4-to-6-Inch) Skewers

BALSAMIC DIPPING SAUCE
- ¼ Cup Olive Oil
- 1 ½ Tbsp Balsamic Vinegar
- 2 Tsp Dijon Mustard
- 2 Tsp Maple Syrup Or Honey
- Pinch of Salt
- Freshly Ground Black Pepper, To Taste

PREPARING THE DISH

1. Onto each skewer, thread the following in alternating patterns: one cherry tomato, one ciliegine, one to two leaves of basil, and a slice of peach or an additional tomato.
2. To prepare the sauce, simply whisk together all of the ingredients in a small bowl until emulsified.
3. Serve skewers on plate with sauce on the side.

PALEO BLUEBERRY MUFFINS

INGREDIENTS

CRUMB TOPPING

- 5 Tbsp Blanched Almond Flour
- 2 Tbsp Refined Coconut Oil (Solid But Soft)
- 3 Tbsp Maple Sugar (Or Coconut Sugar)
- 1 Tsp Cinnamon

MUFFINS

- 4 Large Eggs (Room Temperature)
- ¼ Cup Light Coconut Milk (Room Temperature)
- 1 Tbsp Fresh Lemon Juice (Room Temp)
- 6 Tbsp Maple Sugar (Coconut Sugar)
- 1 Tsp Pure Vanilla Extract
- ½ Tsp Almond Extract (Optional)
- 3 Tbsp Coconut Oil Melted (Cooled To Almost Room Temp)
- 1 ¼ Cups Blanched Almond Flour
- ¼ Cup Coconut Flour
- ¼ Cup Tapioca Flour
- 1 Tsp Baking Soda
- ¼ Tsp Sea Salt
- 2 Tsp Cinnamon
- 1 Cup Fresh Blueberries (You Can Use Frozen If You Thaw And Drain Well Beforehand)

PREPARING THE DISH

1. Preheat your oven to 375° and line a 12 cup muffin pan with parchment liners.

2. Prepare the crumb top first: Place all ingredients together in a medium bowl and combine well using a fork until a thick crumb forms (it will thicken while chilled). Place in the refrigerator while you prepare the muffin batter.

3. Try to have all ingredients at room temperature before

adding. In one bowl, combine the 3 flours, baking soda, salt, and cinnamon. In a separate large bowl, whisk together the eggs, almond milk, lemon juice, sugar, vanilla, almond extract, and coconut oil. I typically add the coconut oil last so it doesn't have time to form solid pieces in the mixture.

4. Once combined, add in the dry mixture and stir (don't vigorously mix or use a blender) until no flour spots can be seen. Lumpy batter is good for the texture and rise of the muffins. Once the dry ingredients are incorporated, gently fold in 3/4 of the blueberries.

5. Spoon the batter into the prepared muffin pan approximately 3/4 of the way full. Top each one with remaining blueberries and a generous sprinkle of the crumb top (I made 12 muffins and used nearly all of the crumb topping).

6. Bake this for 18–20 minutes or until a toothpick inserted in the center of one comes out clean. Allow to cool in the muffin pan for a few minutes before transferring to wire racks to cool completely.

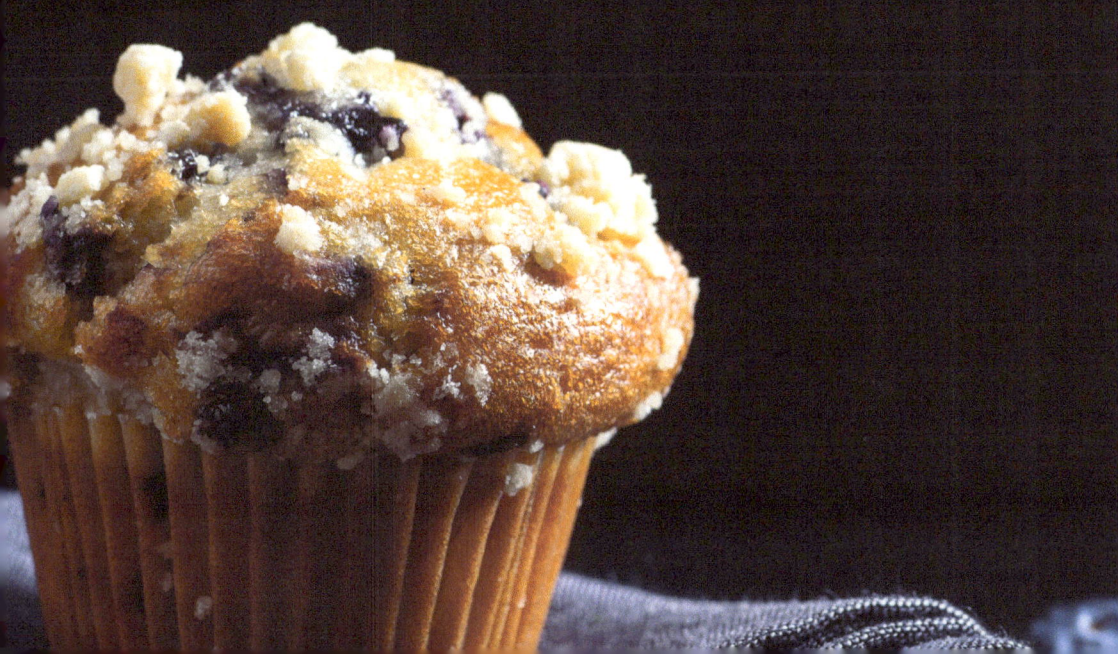

CHICKEN SATAY AND PEANUT SAUCE

INGREDIENTS

CHICKEN
- 1 lb Boneless, Skinless Chicken Breasts, Cut Into 1-Inch Strips
- 2 Tbsp Low-Sodium Soy Sauce Or Tamari For Gluten Free
- ½ Tbsp Fish Sauce Or Additional 1/2 Tbsp Soy Sauce
- 2 Tbsp Freshly Squeezed Lime Juice From 2 Small, Juicy Limes
- 1 Tbsp Honey
- 1 Tbsp Sriracha Sauce
- 2 Tsp Ground Ginger
- 2 Cloves Garlic, Minced

PEANUT SAUCE
- 1 Cup Low Sodium Chicken Broth
- 5 Tbsp Creamy Peanut Butter
- 1 Tbsp Honey
- 1 Tbsp Low-Sodium Soy Sauce Or Tamari For Gluten Free
- 2 Tsp Fish Sauce
- 2 Tsp Sriracha
- 1 Tsp Ground Ginger
- 2 Cloves Garlic, Minced
- 1 Tbsp Freshly Squeezed Lime Juice From 1 Small Lime
- Fresh Cilantro, Chopped
- Unsalted Roasted Peanuts And Lime Wedges For Topping

PREPARING THE DISH

1. In a large mixing bowl, whisk together all of the marinade ingredients, except for the chicken: soy sauce, fish sauce, lime juice, honey, Sriracha, ginger, and garlic. Add the chicken, toss to coat, then cover with plastic wrap and place in the refrigerator to marinate for a minimum of 2 hours. Let stand at room temperature for 30 minutes before grilling. If using wooden skewers, soak the skewers in water for 30 minutes prior to grilling.

2. Meanwhile, prepare the peanut sauce: In a medium saucepan, combine the chicken broth, peanut butter, honey, soy sauce, fish sauce, Sriracha, ginger, and garlic. Bring to a simmer over medium heat, then let cook, stirring often, until the sauce is smooth and has thickened, about 6 minutes. Stir in the lime juice and set aside.

3. When ready to cook, preheat an outdoor grill or indoor grill pan to medium-high. Then thread the chicken onto skewers.

4. Grill chicken until cooked through, about 2–3 minutes per side. Let rest for 2–3 minutes. Sprinkle with peanuts and cilantro, then serve warm with peanut sauce and lime wedges.

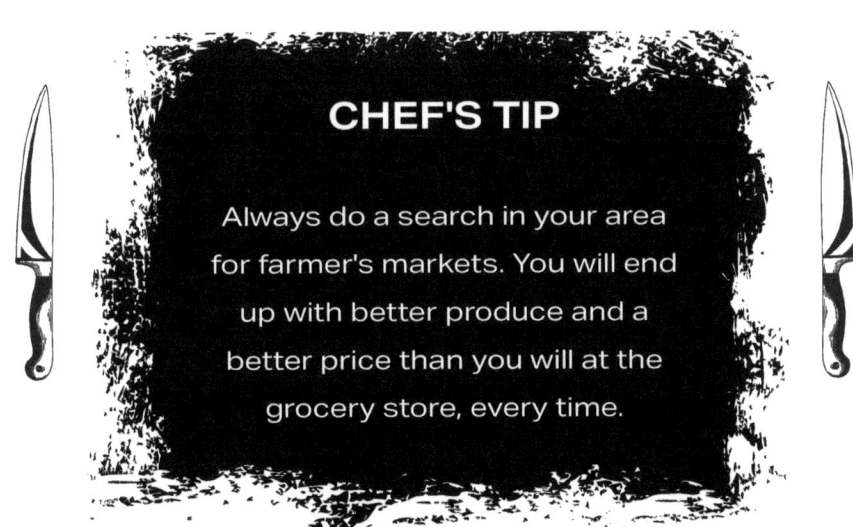

CHEF'S TIP

Always do a search in your area for farmer's markets. You will end up with better produce and a better price than you will at the grocery store, every time.

BAGELS AND LOX (SMOKED SALMON BAGEL)

INGREDIENTS

- 2 Bagels Halved
- 8 Oz Smoked Salmon Thinly Sliced
- 4 Oz Organic Cream Cheese
- 2 Tbsp Lemon Juice
- 1 Tbsp Fresh Dill Plus More For Serving
- Salt and Pepper To Taste
- 1–2 Persian Cucumbers (Or Regular, Peeled In Ribbons)
- Red Onion Slices
- Capers To Taste

PREPARING THE DISH

1. In a small bowl, combine the cream cheese, lemon juice, fresh dill, and salt and pepper to taste.
2. Toast the bagels, then spread the cream cheese mixture on both sides of the bagel. Add the cucumbers, smoked salmon, capers, and red onions onto the bottom half of the toasted bagels. Top with the top of the bagels.

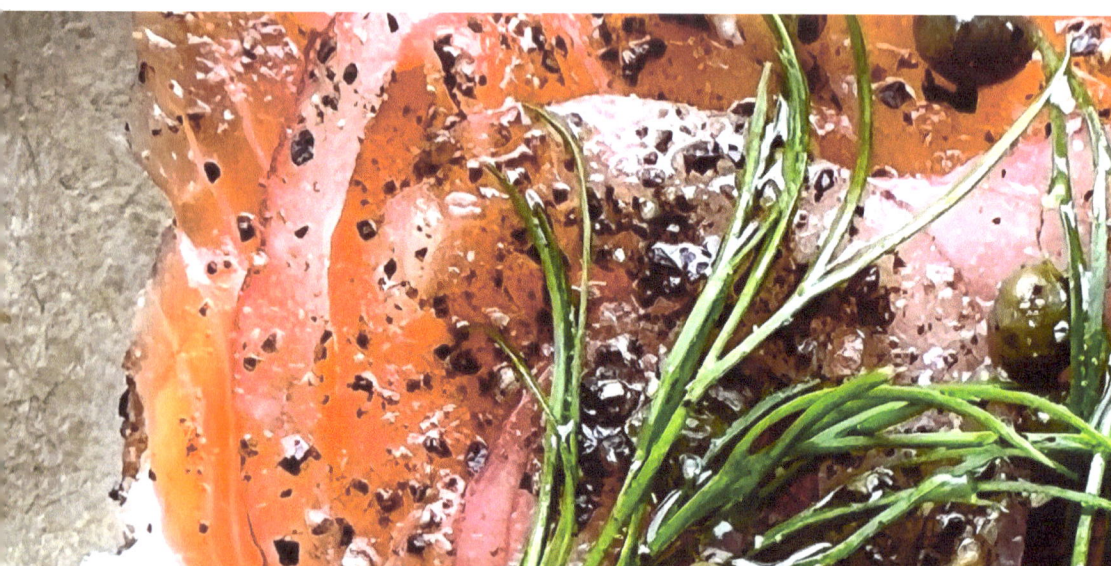

BLUEBERRY COMPOTE PARFAIT

INGREDIENTS

- 1 lb Fresh Or Frozen Blueberries
- 4 Tbsp Fresh Orange Juice
- 4 Tbsp Chia Seeds
- 1 Tbsp Honey
- 1 Cup Greek Yogurt
- ½ Cup Granola
- Optional: Peaches, Mint, Honey or Agave, Nuts

PREPARING THE DISH

1. Add the blueberries and orange juice to a small saucepan on medium heat and let cook for 5–10 minutes, until the liquid begins to evaporate and the blueberries start to thicken. Stir every minute or so to prevent burning. Remove from heat, mix in honey and chia seeds, and let cool completely.
2. Layer the granola, yogurt, blueberry compote, and peach in jars or cups until full. Top with a drizzle of honey and some fresh mint. Makes 2–3 servings.

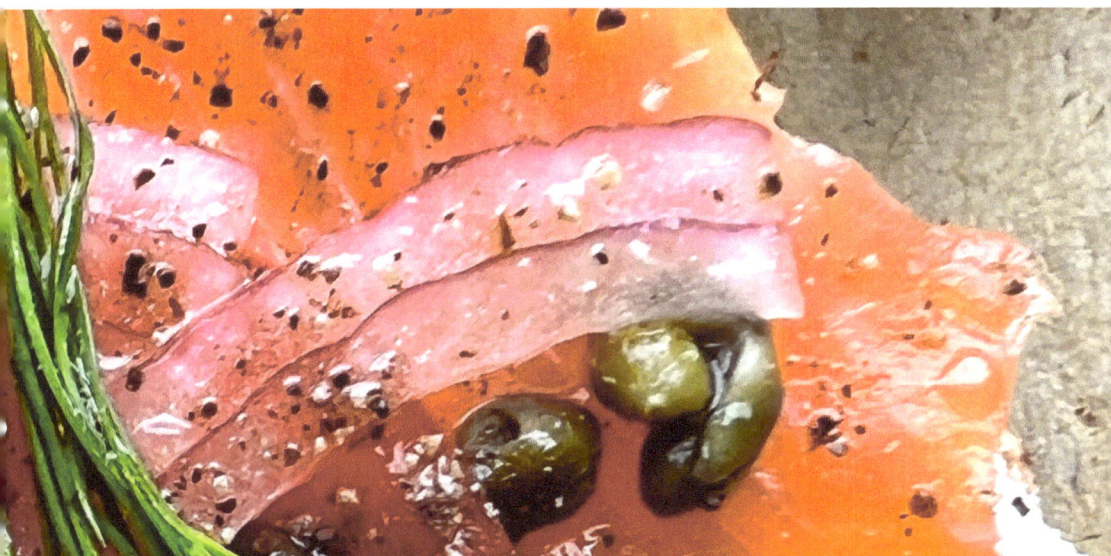

CUCUMBER SALAD

INGREDIENTS

- 1 lb Seedless Cucumbers (Thinly Sliced)
- 1 ½ Tsp Raw Honey
- Pink Himalayan Salt (To Taste)
- 2 ½ Tbsp Rice Wine Vinegar
- 2 Tbsp Scallions (Thinly Sliced)
- 5 Strawberries (Sliced)
- Toasted Sesame Seeds

PREPARING THE DISH

1. In a medium bowl, toss the cucumber slices with the raw honey and salt. Mix in the vinegar, scallions, and strawberries. Refrigerate for 10 minutes. When ready to serve, top with sesame seeds and enjoy

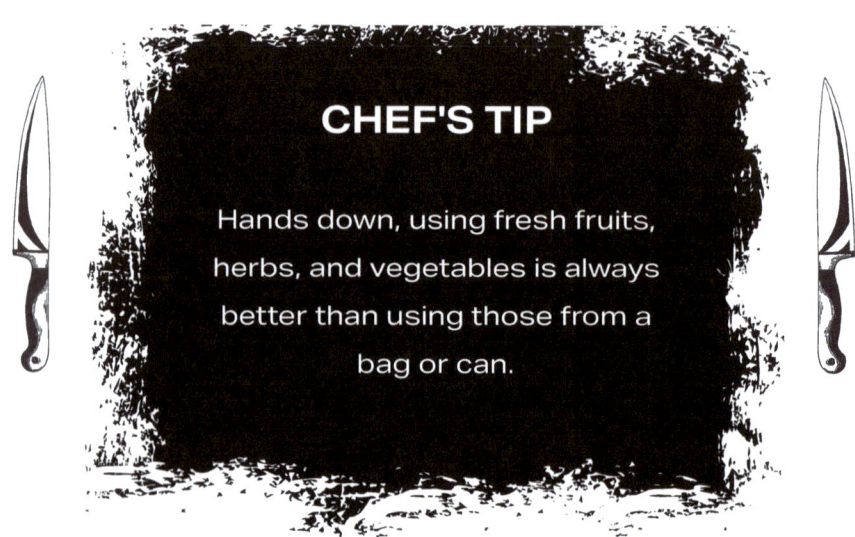

CHEF'S TIP

Hands down, using fresh fruits, herbs, and vegetables is always better than using those from a bag or can.

FRUIT SMOOTHIE

INGREDIENTS

- 1 Ripe Pineapple, Cored And Sliced (About 3 Cups Of Pineapple Chunks)
- 10–12 Mint Leaves, Or To Taste
- 2 Tablespoons Raw Honey, Or To Taste
- 1 ½ Cups Water
- 1 Cup Ice Cubes

PREPARING THE DISH

1. Add all ingredients into a blender and blend until smooth.

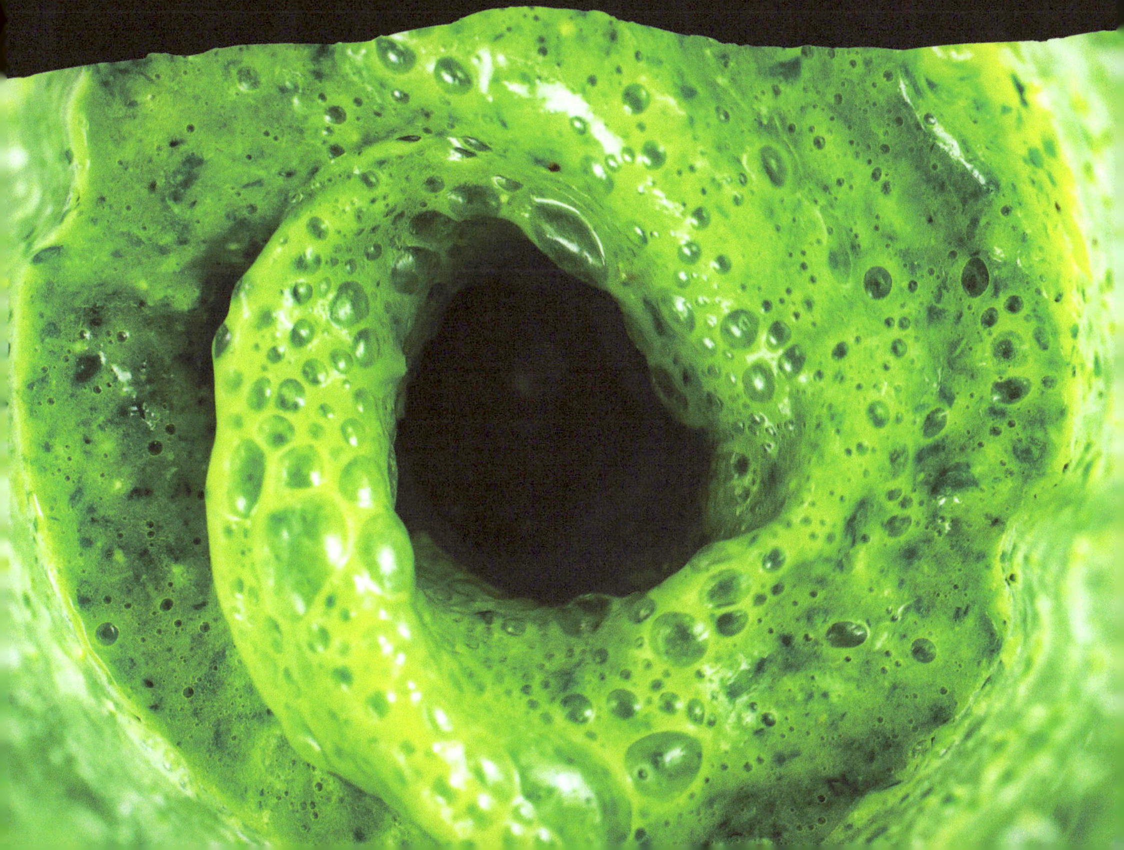

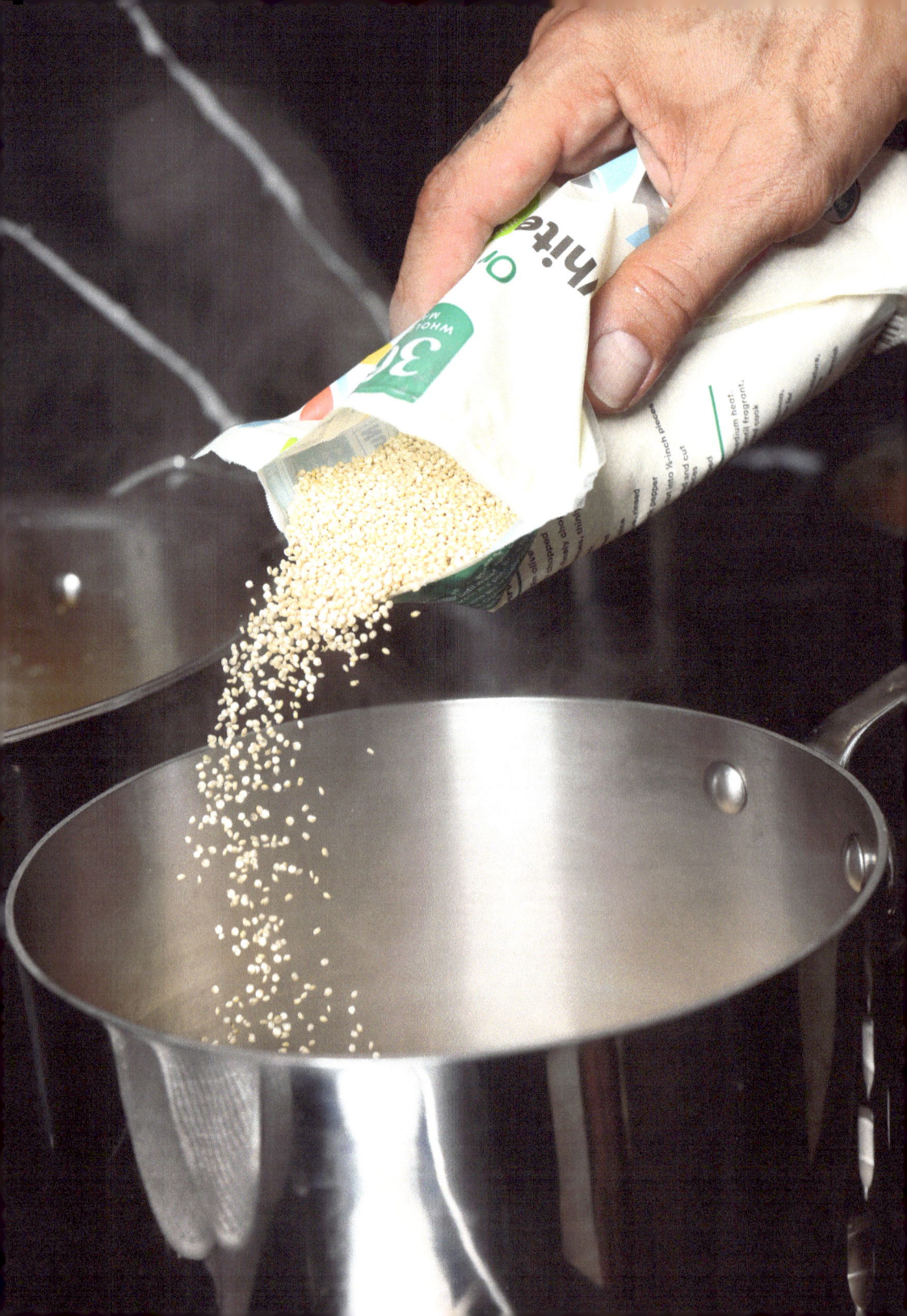

CAULIFLOWER FRIED RICE

INGREDIENTS

- 1 Medium Head of Cauliflower, About 24 Oz, Rinsed
- 1 Tbsp Sesame Oil
- 2 Egg Whites
- 1 Large Egg
- Pinch Of Salt
- Cooking Spray
- ½ Small Onion, Diced Fine
- ½ Cup Frozen Peas and Carrots
- 2 Garlic Cloves, Minced
- 5 Scallions, Diced, Whites and Greens Separated
- 3 Tbsp Soy Sauce, Or More To Taste (Tamari For Gluten Free, Coconut Aminos For Paleo)

PREPARING THE DISH

1. Remove the core and let the cauliflower dry completely.

2. Coarsely chop into florets, then place half of the cauliflower in a food processor and pulse until the cauliflower is small and has the texture of rice or couscous — don't over process, or it will get mushy. Set aside and repeat with the remaining cauliflower.

3. Combine egg and egg whites in a small bowl and beat with a fork. Season with salt.

4. Heat a large saute pan or wok over medium heat and spray with oil. Add the eggs and cook, turning a few times until set; set the cooked eggs aside.

5. Into the pan, add in sesame oil and saute the onions, scallion whites, peas and carrots, and garlic for about 3–4 minutes, or until soft. Raise the heat to medium-high. Add the cauliflower "rice" to the saute pan, along with soy sauce. Mix, cover, and cook approximately 5–6 minutes, stirring frequently, until the cauliflower is slightly crispy on the outside but tender on the inside.

6. Add the egg, then remove from heat and mix in scallion greens.

SPICY ROASTED CHICKPEAS

INGREDIENTS

- 1 Can Organic Chickpeas (Rinsed And Drained)
- 1 Tbsp Extra Virgin Olive Oil
- ½ Tsp Garlic Powder
- 2 Tsp Chili Powder
- ¼ Tsp Pink Himalayan Salt
- 1 Tbsp Chives (Finely Chopped)
- 1 Lime's Finely Grated Lime Zest

PREPARING THE DISH

1. Rinse chickpeas and dry with paper towels. Let them sit for 15 minutes, then dry again. In a medium bowl, toss chickpeas, oil, chili powder, garlic powder, and salt. Make sure to coat them well.

2. Transfer chickpea mixture to an air-fryer basket, scraping the bowl to get all of the oil. Cook at 370° until crispy and golden brown, 10–14 minutes. You can use convect bake on your oven if you do not have an air fryer.

3. Grate lime zest and sprinkle chives over top. Then plate and serve.

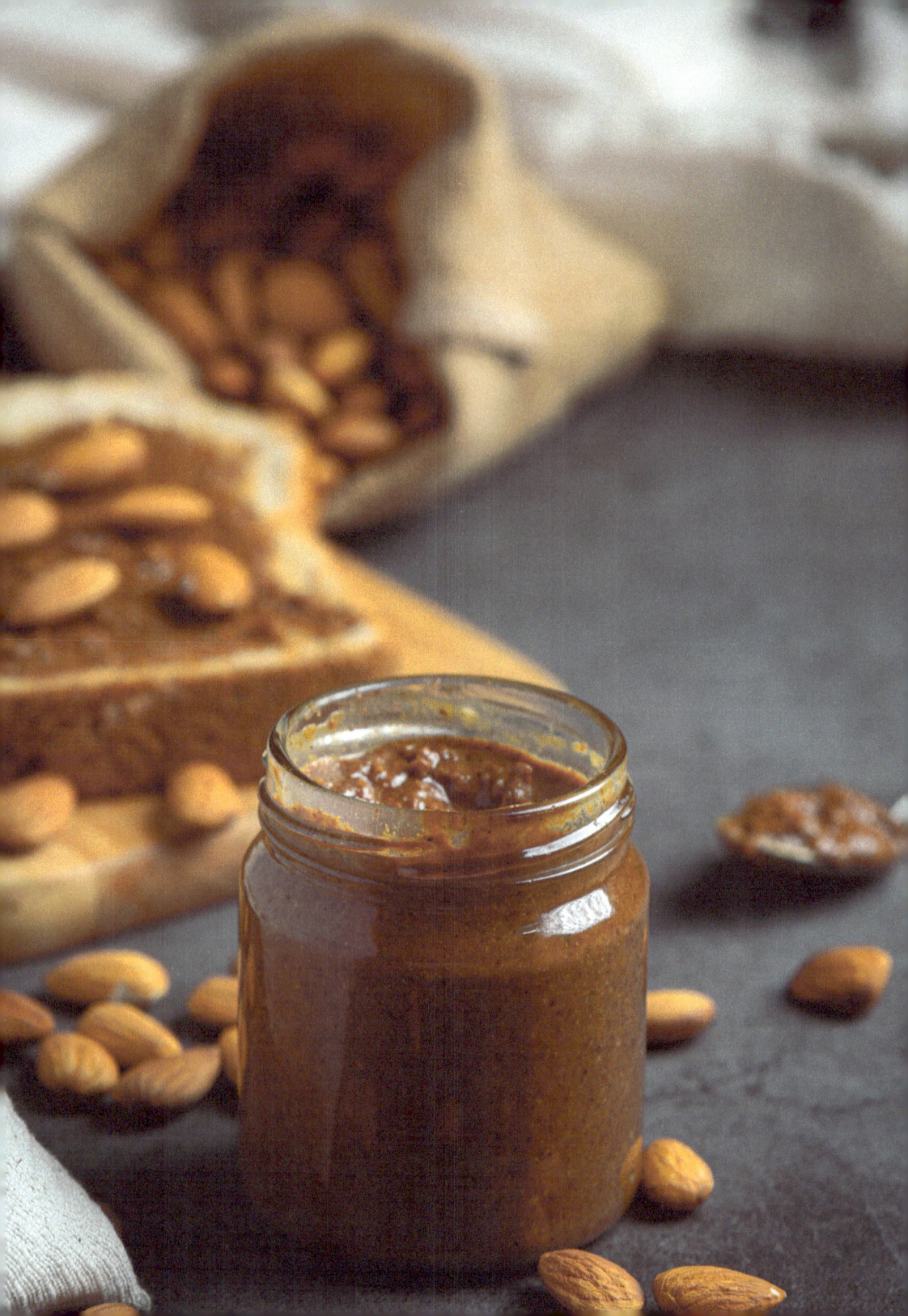

ALMOND BUTTER BALLS

INGREDIENTS

- 1 Cup Old Fashioned Rolled Oats
- ½ Cup Almond Butter
- ⅓ Cup Honey
- 2 Tbsp Chocolate Protein Powder
- Shredded Coconut (Optional)

PREPARING THE DISH

1. Combine all ingredients in a blender or food processor until completely smooth. Split in 4 portions and chill.

AVOCADO CHOCOLATE MOUSSE

INGREDIENTS

- Flesh Of 2 Ripe Avocados
- 1/4 Cup Regular Cocoa Powder
- 1/4 Cup Dutch Cocoa Or Melted Organic Chocolate Chips
- 3-4 Tbsp Milk Of Choice
- 1/2 Tsp Pure Vanilla Extract
- Salt To Taste
- 1/4 Cup Pure Maple Syrup (Or Sweetener Of Choice)

PREPARING THE DISH

1. Combine everything in your food processor and blend until thick and smooth.

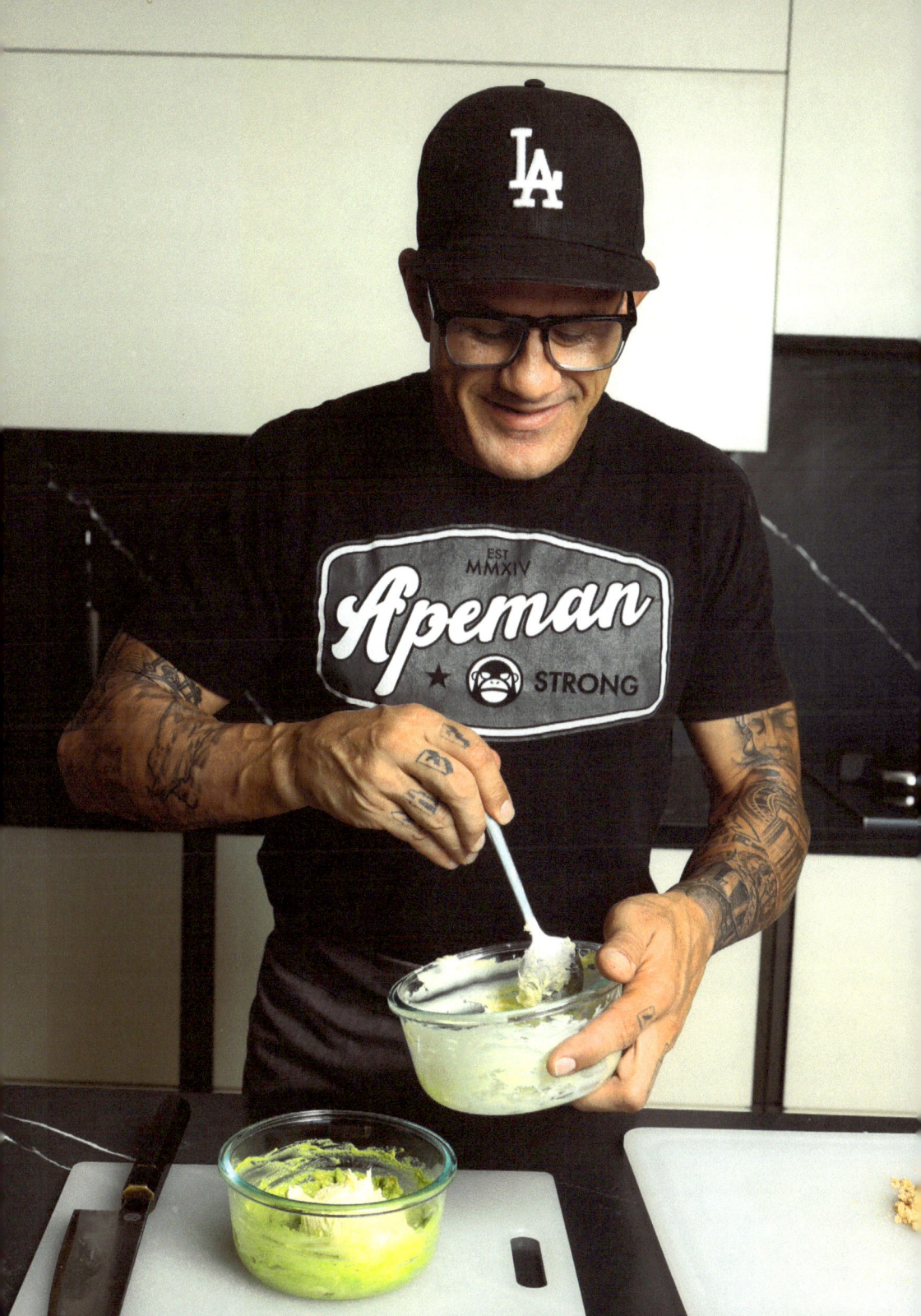

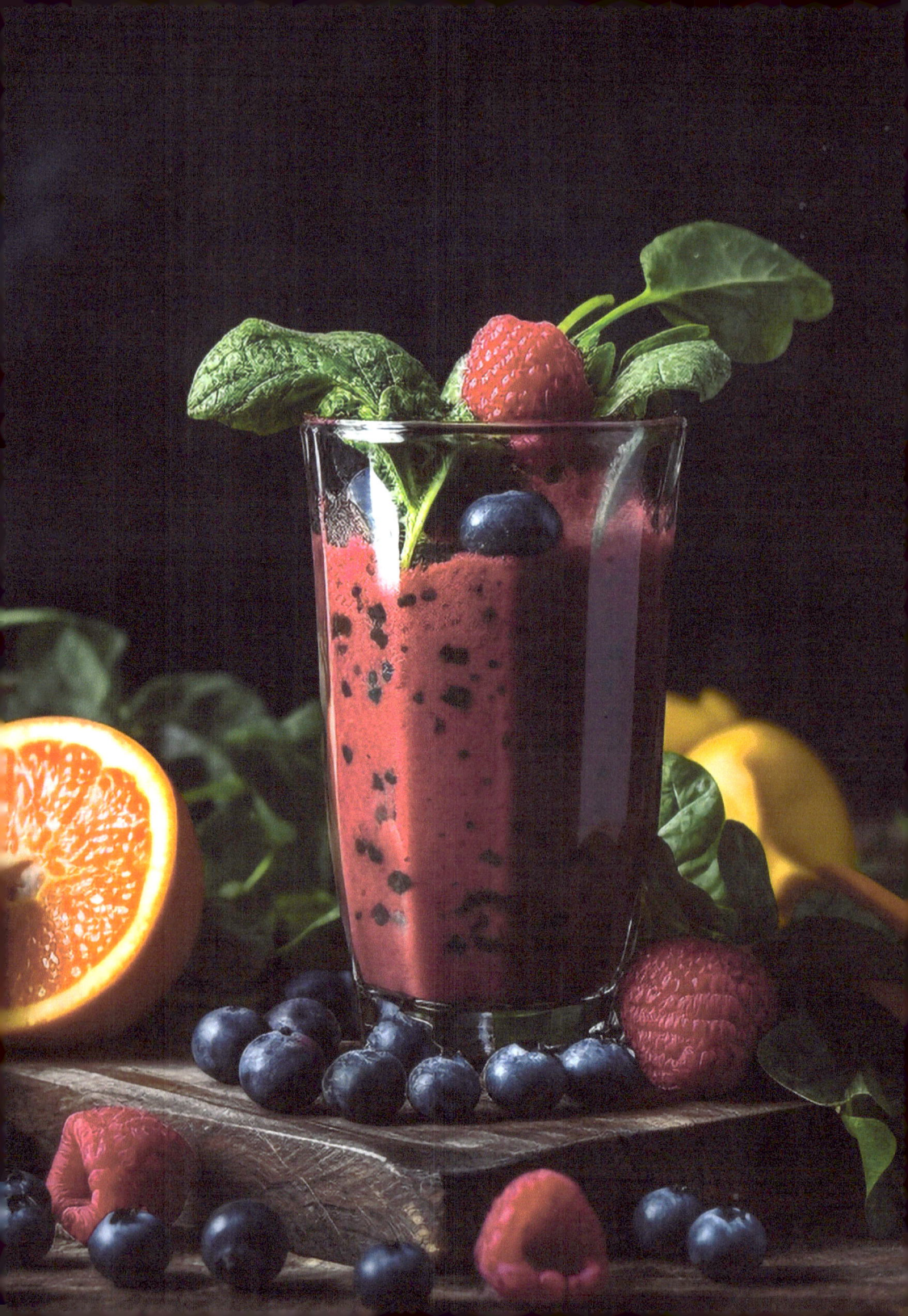

SMOOTHIES

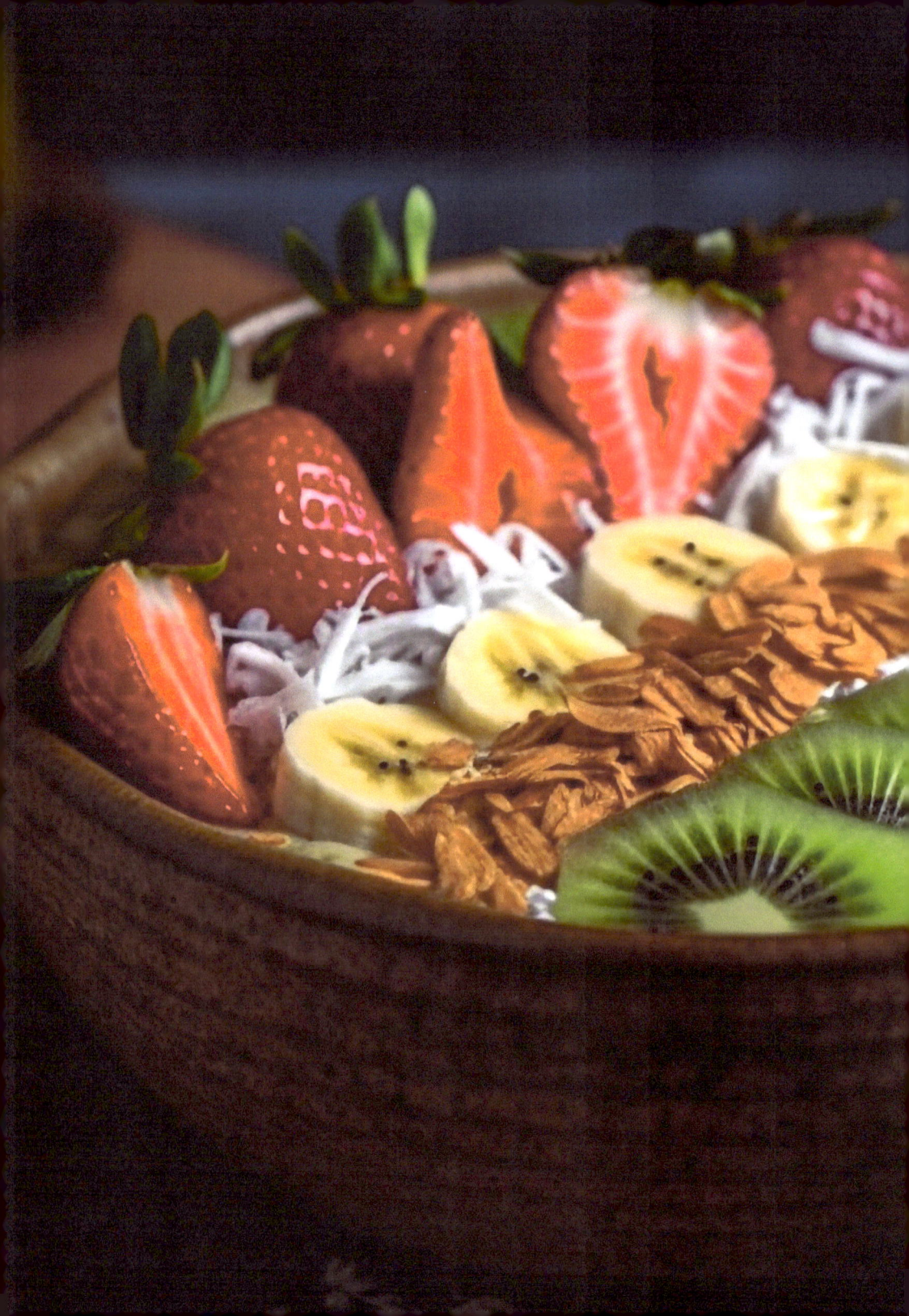

GREEN SMOOTHIE BOWL

INGREDIENTS

- 1 Frozen Banana
- 1 Avocado
- 2 Cups Spinach
- 1 Apple
- ¼ Cup Almond Milk
- ½ Cup Ice
- 2 Tbsp Goji Berries
- 2 Tbsp Toasted Coconut
- 1 Tbsp Chopped Macadamia Nuts
- 1 Sliced Kiwi

PREPARING THE DISH

1. In a blender, combine banana, avocado, spinach, apple, almond milk, and ice; blend until smooth. Pour the smoothie into a bowl and garnish with goji berries, toasted coconut, chopped macadamia nuts, and sliced kiwi.

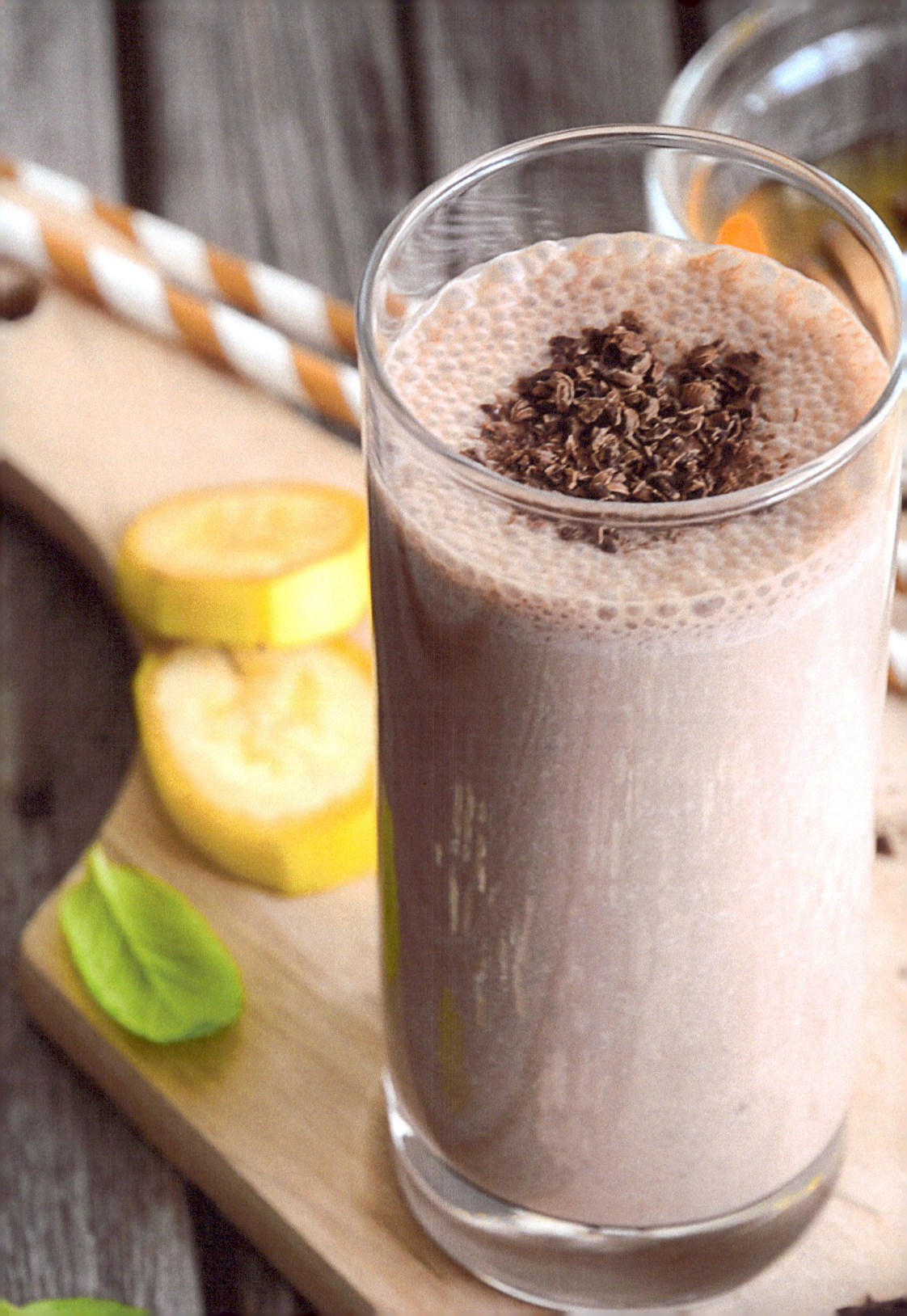

COCOA ALMOND PROTEIN SMOOTHIE

INGREDIENTS

- ¾ Cup Greek Yogurt
- ¼ Cup Plus 2 Tbsp Milk
- 1 Medium Banana, Sliced And Frozen
- ½ Tablespoon Unsweetened Cocoa Powder
- 2 Tablespoons Almond Butter
- 2 Teaspoon Ground Flaxseed, Optional
- ¾ Cup Ice Cubes

PREPARING THE DISH

1. Add all ingredients into a blender and blend until smooth.

OATMEAL BREAKFAST SMOOTHIE

INGREDIENTS

- ¼ Cup Old-Fashioned Oats Or Quick Oats
- 1 Banana Chopped Into Chunks And Frozen
- ½ Cup Unsweetened Almond Milk
- 1 Tbsp Creamy Peanut Butter
- ½ Tbsp Pure Maple Syrup Plus Additional To Taste
- ½ Tsp Pure Vanilla Extract
- ½ Tsp Ground Cinnamon
- ⅛ Tsp Kosher Salt (Don't Skip This, As It Makes The Oatmeal Pop!)
- Ice (Optional For A Thicker Smoothie)

PREPARING THE DISH

1. Place the oats in the bottom of a blender and pulse a few times until finely ground. Add the banana, milk, peanut butter, maple syrup, vanilla, cinnamon, and salt. Blend until smooth and creamy, stopping to scrape down the blender as needed. Taste and add additional sweetener if you'd like a sweeter smoothie.

REHYDRATION SMOOTHIE

INGREDIENTS

- 2 Cups Baby Spinach
- 2 Cups Chopped Pineapple
- 1 Medium Banana
- 1 Cup Coconut Almond Milk Blend
- 1 Cup Ice Cubes

PREPARING THE DISH

1. Add all ingredients into a blender and blend until smooth.

CARAMEL PROTEIN SHAKE

INGREDIENTS

- 1 Cup Milk
- ¼ Cup Chickpeas Drained And Rinse
- 1 Tbsp Cashew Butter
- 2–3 Medjool Dates Pitted
- 2 Tsp Coconut Sugar
- 1 Cup Ice

PREPARING THE DISH

1. Blend chickpeas, dates, and milk until smooth. Scrape down sides and blend again if needed. Add cashew butter and coconut sugar and blend again until smooth. Pour over a glass of ice and enjoy!

CHOCOLATE COVERED STRAWBERRY SMOOTHIE

INGREDIENTS

- 1 Cup Milk Or Milk Alternative
- 1 Cup Frozen Strawberries
- 2 Dates
- 3 Cups Baby Spinach
- 2 Scoops Chocolate Protein Powder
- 1 Avocado

PREPARING THE DISH

1. Add all ingredients into a blender and blend until smooth.

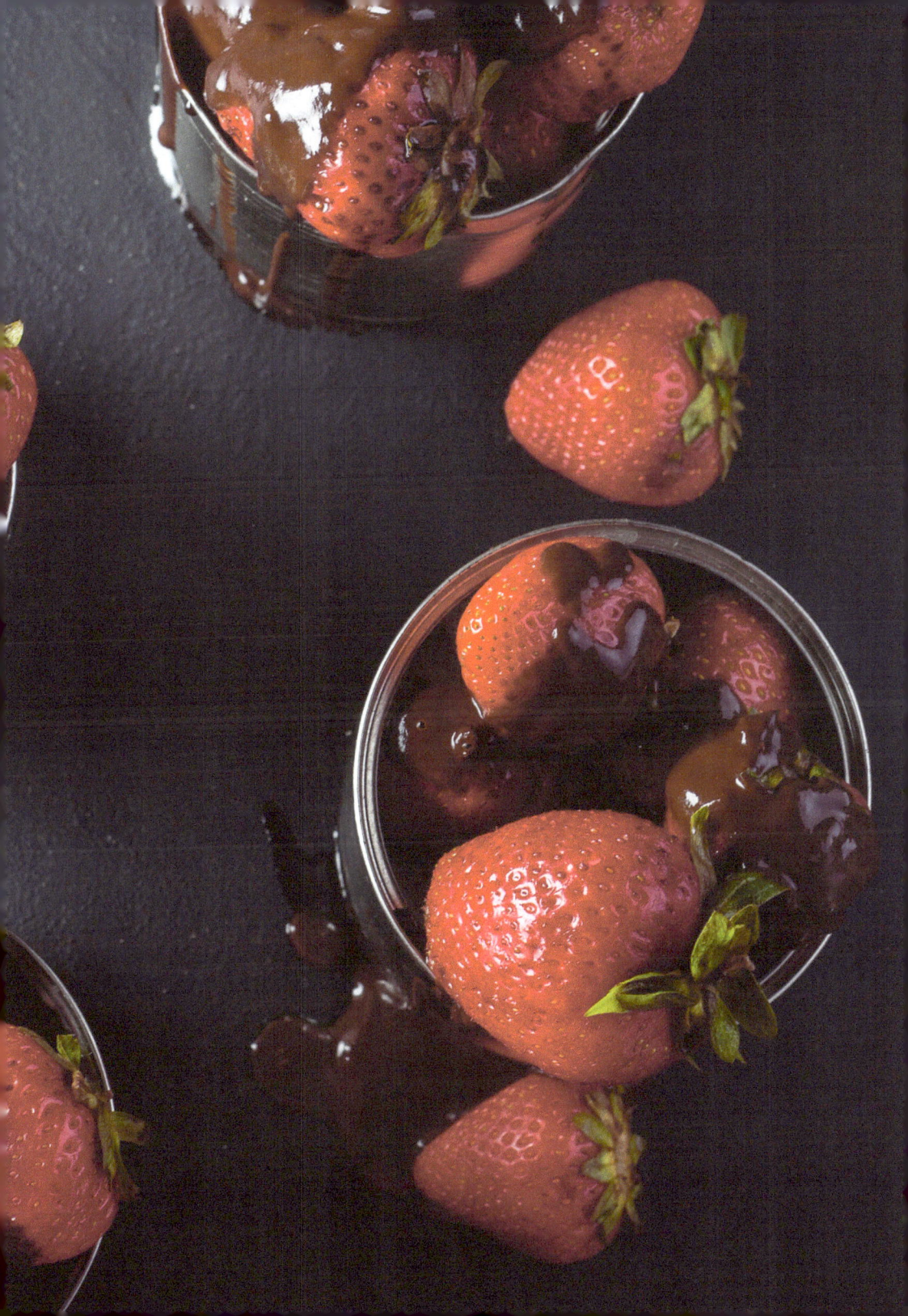

CUT WEIGHT QUICK LIKE A PRO

1. Setting goals and having a plan are very important when it comes to losing or cutting weight. This will give you a clear line of sight on what needs to be achieved. You are more likely to stay on track. So set goals, have a plan, and write it all down.
2. Monitor your calorie intake so you know what you are consuming.
3. Meal prepping and planning your meals is important, and allows an easier way to monitor your calories. When you meal prep and plan meals out, you eliminate the probability of missing a meal. You can also plan out exactly what you need to eat to reach your goals.
4. Make sure you are at a caloric deficit, which means that you are burning more calories than you are consuming.
5. Daily activity and workouts are super important to losing weight. Certain workouts help us burn fat. Working out will also help burn more calories, which will keep us in that caloric deficit.
6. Stick to high-quality foods and ingredients, as high-quality food and ingredients allow for better body function)
7. Make sure you are getting plenty of sleep. Getting the right amount of sleep will allow the body to rest and recover.
8. Drink enough water. Drinking the right amount of water will keep you hydrated, keep your organs functioning properly, and actually help with maintaining weight.
9. If you need to lose a quick few pounds quickly, you can do a sauna. This is only water weight loss, and you will gain it back when you rehydrate.

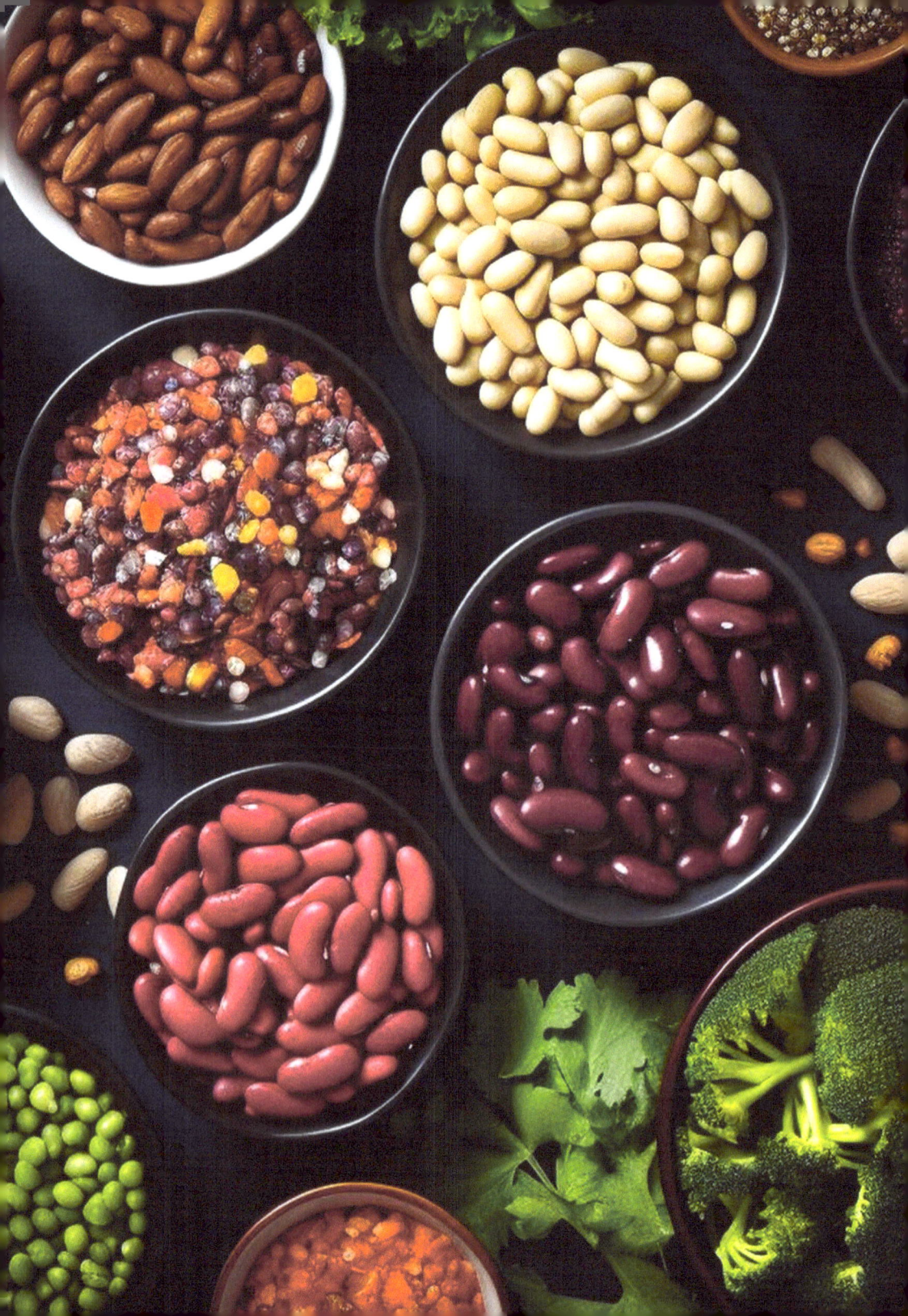

MACROS

	RECIPE	CALORIES	CARBS (g)	*	%
					MAIN MEALS
1	SHRIMP AND GARLIC PASTA	1810	150	600	33%
2	AVOCADO CHICKEN SALAD SANDWICH	533	17	68	13%
3	CHICKEN PASTA SALAD	791	91	364	46%
4	SALMON POKE	450	55	220	49%
5	PAN SEARED SALMON AND VEGGIES	675	41	164	24%
6	BROCCOLI WITH BEEF	322	24	96	30%
7	ORANGE CHICKEN OVER QUINOA	1241	132	528	43%
8	TURKEY CHILI	741	88	352	48%
9	SALMON CAKES	609	65	260	43%
10	QUINOA SQUASH SALAD	963	92	368	38%
11	STEAK EGGS CHILE VERDE	1039	10	40	4%
12	LASAGNA	1460	112	448	31%
					SIGNATURE DISHES
1	DEMI LOVATO CHEESECAKE	1312	71	284	22%
2	KSI COD	405	55	220	54%
3	LOGAN PAUL BUTTER NOODLES	714	85	340	48%
4	DK SALMON	419	26	104	25%
5	CONORS LAMB CHOPS	563	43	172	31%
6	PATRICKS CURRY	416	13	52	13%
					BREAKFASTS
1	EGG SCRAMBLE	671	19	76	11%
2	POTATO FRITATTA	520	27	108	21%
3	EVERYTHING BAGEL SALMON	577	8	32	6%
4	EGG SCRAMBLE SIMPLE	357	34	136	38%
5	EGG GOAT CHEESE SCRAMBLE	422	13	52	12%
6	AVOCADO TOAST	357	33	132	37%
7	CREPES	379	46	184	49%
8	FRIED EGG SANDWICH	537	43	172	32%
9	BANANA PANCAKES	632	94	376	59%
					SNACKS
1	OVERNIGHT CHIA CUPS	858	98	392	46%
2	CAPRESE SLIDERS	289	1.5	6	2%
3	PALEO BLUEBERRY MUFFINS	2620	133	532	20%
4	CHICKEN SATAY	750	25	100	13%
5	BAGELS AND LOX	1286	161	644	50%
6	BLUEBERRY COMPOTE PARFAIT	995	191	764	77%
7	CUCUMBER SALAD	160	32	128	80%
8	FRUIT SMOOTHIE	380	90	360	95%
9	CAULIFLOWER FRIED RICE	243	24	96	40%
10	SPICY ROASTED CHICKPEAS	270	32	128	47%
11	ALMOND BUTTER BALLS	375	31	124	33%
12	AVOCADO CHOCOLATE MOUSSE	511	56	224	44%

PROTEIN (g)	*	%	FAT (g)	*	%	FORMULA CHECK
120	480	27%	80.5	725	40%	100%
38	152	29%	35	315	59%	100%
39	156	20%	30	270	34%	100%
35	140	31%	10	90	20%	100%
42	168	25%	38	342	51%	100%
28	112	35%	12.5	113	35%	100%
96	384	31%	36	324	26%	100%
79	316	43%	8	72	10%	100%
49	196	32%	17	153	25%	100%
41	164	17%	48	432	45%	100%
53	212	20%	88	792	76%	100%
105	420	29%	66	594	41%	100%
10	40	3%	110	990	75%	100%
15	60	15%	14	126	31%	100%
33	132	18%	27	243	34%	100%
50	200	48%	13	117	28%	100%
37	148	26%	27	243	43%	100%
30	120	29%	27	243	58%	100%
52	208	31%	43	387	58%	100%
31	124	24%	32	288	55%	100%
58	232	40%	35	315	55%	100%
24	96	27%	14	126	35%	100%
20	80	19%	32	288	68%	100%
24	96	27%	14.5	131	37%	100%
17	68	18%	14	126	33%	100%
33	132	25%	26	234	44%	100%
17	68	11%	21	189	30%	100%
24	96	11%	41	369	43%	100%
23.57	94.3	33%	21	189	65%	100%
246	984	38%	124	1116	43%	100%
53	212	28%	49	441	59%	100%
72	288	22%	40	360	28%	100%
25	100	10%	15	135	14%	100%
2	8	5%	2.7	24.3	15%	100%
3	12	3%	1	9	2%	100%
14	56	23%	10	90	37%	100%
11	44	16%	11	99	37%	100%
11	44	12%	23	207	55%	100%
9	36	7%	28	252	49%	100%

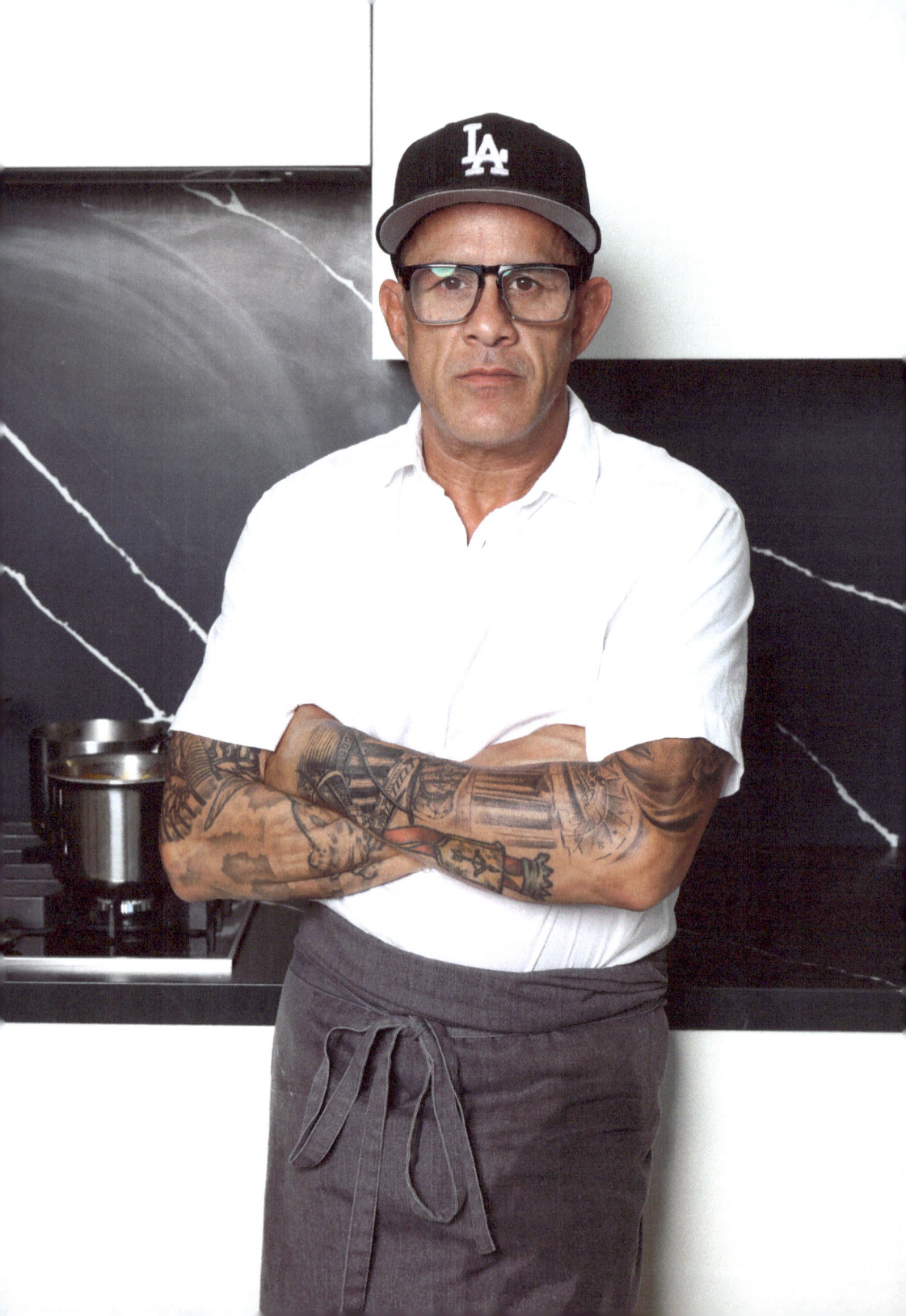

THANK YOU

Thank you to all the people who have helped me along my journey:

My mom, for your strength and sacrifices while raising me on your own, and for always loving me, no matter what.

Alyssa Daley Phillips, because I wouldn't have gotten it done without your help.

I want to thank all the fighters who have trusted me with their health, and with getting them on weight safely.

Conor, thanks for all the good times and great memories.

Logan, thanks for trusting me with your weight cuts for some historical fights.

Thank you to my daughter, Caprese. You give me motivation to do better and be better every day.

Finally, thank you to Sequoia and the team at DAP for making it all happen.

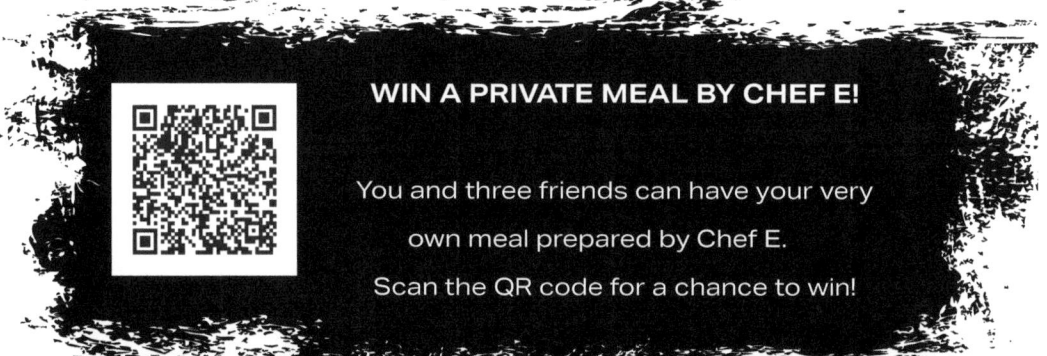

WIN A PRIVATE MEAL BY CHEF E!

You and three friends can have your very own meal prepared by Chef E. Scan the QR code for a chance to win!

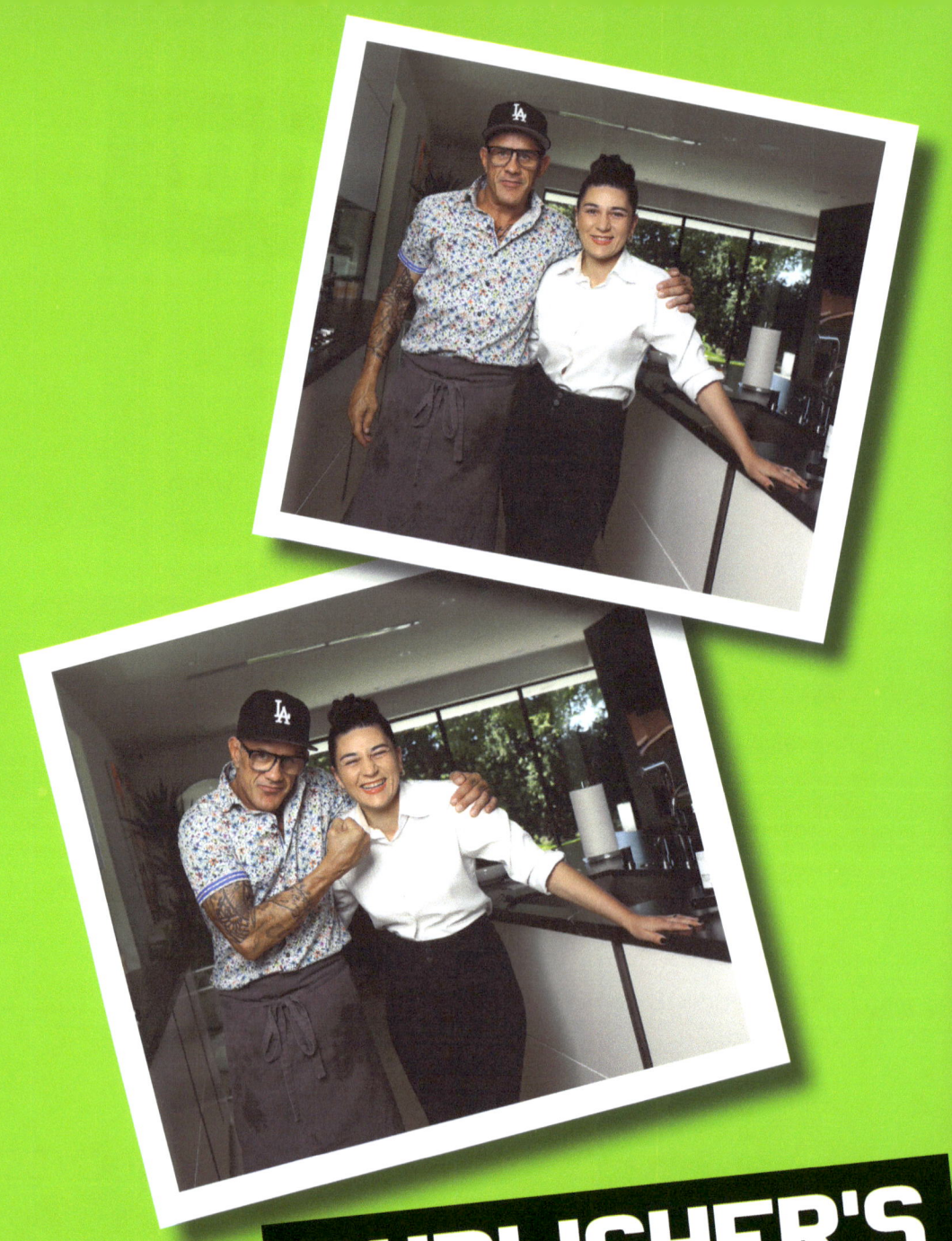

PUBLISHER'S NOTE

When Eric first mentioned the idea of doing a cookbook, I was immediately intrigued. I knew that Eric worked with a number of big clients, and seemed to be well respected and genuinely liked in his field. For the most part, my job is to find the story, and with Eric, there was a natural question of "How." How did you go from a small-town line cook to being the personal chef to some of the top fighters in the world? What's more than that, is the question: How have you stayed so humble and grounded through the process of your success?

For those of you who don't know Eric personally, he's grounded. Grounded in a way that is rare for someone who has achieved his level of success, working with some of the biggest names in the world. I knew it from the moment I first met him, there was a genuine coolness to his demeanor that made me want to get to know him further, that made me intrigued to jump on a project when it was pitched to me.

During our first Zoom about the book, Eric was at Logan Paul's house as Logan was preparing for an upcoming fight. Eric began pitching me on the idea of a cookbook. He obviously knew his craft in the kitchen, or he wouldn't be working with these guys, but I knew his story was too interesting to just do a pamphlet of recipes.

To be honest, it wasn't until the photoshoot many months later that I really understood the level of Eric's skill. One of the fun parts about doing a book like this is eating all the food after it is photographed. By the time we were shooting, I already knew all the stories behind each dish. Through a series of interviews, Eric divulged how each recipe came to be and which fighter liked which dish. Eric is a busy man, so it took a lot from us to pull this book together in a way that myself and my team were happy with.

I remember sorting through layout with my artistic director for the publishing firm — and thinking about how cool this project was. Drawing inspirations from other kickass cookbooks like "Thug Kitchen," while simultaneously implementing some of the stories behind the dishes, and autobiographical elements. I wanted the book to be raw and grungy, capturing the fight world and the struggle Eric went through to get to where he is today.

I hope that this will be the first of many books to come with Eric, and I'm excited about what the future has to offer.

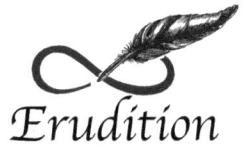

ABOUT THE PUBLISHER

Di Angelo Publications was founded in 2008 by Sequoia Schmidt—at the age of seventeen. The modernized publishing firm's creative headquarters is in Los Angeles, California, with its distribution center located in Twin Falls, Idaho. In 2020, Di Angelo Publications made a conscious decision to move all printing and production for domestic distribution of its books to the United States. The firm is comprised of eleven imprints, and the featured imprint, Erudition, was inspired by the desire to spread knowledge, spark curiosity, and add numbers to the ranks of continuing learners, big and small.

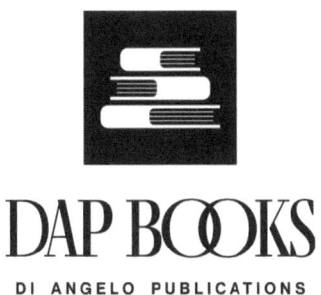

www.ingramcontent.com/pod-product-compliance
Lightning Source LLC
Chambersburg PA
CBHW042016150426
43197CB00002B/40